Cleborne D. Maddux
D. LaMont Johnson
Editors

The Web in Higher Education: Assessing the Impact and Fulfilling the Potential

The Web in Higher Education: Assessing the Impact and Fulfilling the Potential has been co-published simultaneously as *Computers in the Schools*, Volume 17, Numbers 3/4 and Volume 18, Number 1 2001.

*Pre-publication
REVIEWS,
COMMENTARIES,
EVALUATIONS . . .*

"I ENTHUSIASTICALLY RECOMMEND THIS BOOK to anyone new to Web-based program development. I am certain that my project has moved along more rapidly because of what I learned from this text. The chapter on designing online education courses helped to organize my programmatic thinking. Another chapter did an outstanding job of debunking the myths regarding Web learning."

Carol Swift, PhD
*Associate Professor and Chair
of the Department of Human Development
and Child Studies,
Oakland University, Rochester, Michigan*

More pre-publication
REVIEWS, COMMENTARIES, EVALUATIONS . . .

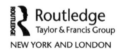
Routledge
Taylor & Francis Group

NEW YORK AND LONDON

The Web in Higher Education:
Assessing the Impact
and Fulfilling the Potential

The Web in Higher Education: Assessing the Impact and Fulfilling the Potential has been co-published simultaneously as *Computers in the Schools,* Volume 17, Numbers 3/4 and Volume 18, Number 1 2001.

The *Computers in the Schools* Monographic "Separates"

Below is a list of "separates," which in serials librarianship means a special issue simultaneously published as a special journal issue or double-issue *and* as a "separate" hardbound monograph. (This is a format which we also call a "DocuSerial.")

"Separates" are published because specialized libraries or professionals may wish to purchase a specific thematic issue by itself in a format which can be separately cataloged and shelved, as opposed to purchasing the journal on an on-going basis. Faculty members may also more easily consider a "separate" for classroom adoption.

"Separates" are carefully classified separately with the major book jobbers so that the journal tie-in can be noted on new book order slips to avoid duplicate purchasing.

You may wish to visit Haworth's website at . . .

http://www.HaworthPress.com

. . . to search our online catalog for complete tables of contents of these separates and related publications.

You may also call 1-800-HAWORTH (outside US/Canada: 607-722-5857), or Fax 1-800-895-0582 (outside US/Canada: 607-771-0012), or e-mail at:

getinfo@haworthpressinc.com

The Web in Higher Education: Assessing the Impact and Fulfilling the Potential, edited by Cleborne D. Maddux, PhD, and D. LaMont Johnson, PhD (Vol. 17, No. 3/4 and Vol. 18, No. 1, 2001). *"I ENTHUSIASTICALLY RECOMMEND THIS BOOK to anyone new to Web-based program development. I am certain that my project has moved along more rapidly because of what I learned from this text. The chapter on designing online education courses helped to organize my programmatic thinking. Another chapter did an outstanding job of debunking the myths regarding Web learning."* (Carol Swift, PhD, Associate Professor and Chair of the Department of Human Development and Child Studies, Oakland University, Rochester, Michigan)

Using Information Technology in Mathematics Education, edited by D. James Tooke, PhD, and Norma Henderson, MS (Vol. 17, No. 1/2 2001). *"Provides thought-provoking material on several aspects and levels of mathematics education. The ideas presented will provide food for thought for the reader, suggest new methods for the classroom, and give new ideas for further research."* (Charles E. Lamb, EdD, Professor, Mathematics Education, Department of Teaching, Learning, and Culture, College of Education, Texas A&M University, College Station)

Integration of Technology into the Classroom: Case Studies, edited by D. LaMont Johnson, PhD, Cleborne D. Maddux, PhD, and Leping Liu, PhD (Vol. 16, No. 2/3/4, 2000). *Use these fascinating case studies to understand why bringing information technology into your classroom can make you a more effective teacher, and how to go about it!*

Information Technology in Educational Research and Statistics, edited by Leping Liu, PhD, D. LaMont Johnson, PhD, and Cleborne D. Maddux, PhD (Vol. 15, No. 3/4, and Vol. 16, No. 1, 1999). *This important book focuses on creating new ideas for using educational technologies such as the Internet, the World Wide Web and various software packages to further research and statistics. You will explore on-going debates relating to the theory of research, research methodology, and successful practices.* Information Technology in Educational Research and Statistics *also covers the debate on what statistical procedures are appropriate for what kinds of research designs.*

Educational Computing in the Schools: Technology, Communication, and Literacy, edited by Jay Blanchard, PhD (Vol. 15, No. 1, 1999). *Examines critical issues of technology, teaching, and learning in three areas: access, communication, and literacy. You will discover new ideas and practices for gaining access to and using technology in education from preschool through higher education.*

Logo: A Retrospective, edited by Cleborne D. Maddux, PhD, and D. LaMont Johnson, PhD (Vol. 14, No. 1/2, 1997). *"This book–honest and optimistic–is a must for those interested in any aspect of*

Logo: its history, the effects of its use, or its general role in education." (Dorothy M. Fitch, Logo consultant, writer, and editor, Derry, New Hampshire)

Using Technology in the Classroom, edited by D. LaMont Johnson, PhD, Cleborne D. Maddux, PhD, and Leping Liu, MS (Vol. 13, No. 1/2, 1997). *"A guide to teaching with technology that emphasizes the advantages of transiting from teacher-directed learning to learner-centered learning–a shift that can draw in even 'at-risk' kids." (Book News, Inc.)*

Multimedia and Megachange: New Roles for Educational Computing, edited by W. Michael Reed, PhD, John K. Burton, PhD, and Min Liu, EdD (Vol. 10, No. 1/2/3/4, 1995). *"Describes and analyzes issues and trends that might set research and development agenda for educators in the near future." (Sci Tech Book News)*

Language Minority Students and Computers, edited by Christian J. Faltis, PhD, and Robert A. DeVillar, PhD (Vol. 7, No. 1/2, 1990). *"Professionals in the field of language minority education, including ESL and bilingual education, will cheer this collection of articles written by highly respected, research-writers, along with computer technologists, and classroom practitioners." (Journal of Computing in Teacher Education)*

Logo: Methods and Curriculum for Teachers, by Cleborne D. Maddux, PhD, and D. LaMont Johnson, PhD (Supp #3, 1989). *"An excellent introduction to this programming language for children." (Rena B. Lewis, Professor, College of Education, San Diego State University)*

Assessing the Impact of Computer-Based Instruction: A Review of Recent Research, by M. D. Roblyer, PhD, W. H. Castine, PhD, and F. J. King, PhD (Vol. 5, No. 3/4, 1988). *"A comprehensive and up-to-date review of the effects of computer applications on student achievement and attitudes." (Measurements & Control)*

Educational Computing and Problem Solving, edited by W. Michael Reed, PhD, and John K. Burton, PhD (Vol. 4, No. 3/4, 1988). *Here is everything that educators will need to know to use computers to improve higher level skills such as problem solving and critical thinking.*

The Computer in Reading and Language Arts, edited by Jay S. Blanchard, PhD, and George E. Mason, PhD (Vol. 4, No. 1, 1987). *"All of the [chapters] in this collection are useful, guiding the teacher unfamiliar with classroom computer use through a large number of available software options and classroom strategies." (Educational Technology)*

Computers in the Special Education Classroom, edited by D. LaMont Johnson, PhD, Cleborne D. Maddux, PhD, and Ann Candler, PhD (Vol. 3, No. 3/4, 1987). *"A good introduction to the use of computers in special education. . . . Excellent for those who need to become familiar with computer usage with special population students because they are contemplating it or because they have actually just begun to do it." (Science Books and Films)*

You Can Do It/Together, by Kathleen A. Smith, PhD, Cleborne D. Maddux, PhD, and D. LaMont Johnson, PhD (Supp #2, 1986). *A self-instructional textbook with an emphasis on the partnership system of learning that introduces the reader to four critical areas of computer technology.*

Computers and Teacher Training: A Practical Guide, by Dennis M. Adams, PhD (Supp #1, 1986). *"A very fine . . . introduction to computer applications in education." (International Reading Association)*

The Computer as an Educational Tool, edited by Henry F. Olds, Jr. (Vol. 3, No. 1, 1986). *"The category of tool uses for computers holds the greatest promise for learning, and this . . . book, compiled from the experiences of a good mix of practitioners and theorists, explains how and why." (Jack Turner, Technology Coordinator, Eugene School District 4-J, Oregon)*

Logo in the Schools, edited by Cleborne D. Maddux, PhD (Vol. 2, No. 2/3, 1985). *"An excellent blend of enthusiasm for the language of Logo mixed with empirical analysis of the language's effectiveness as a means of promoting educational goals. A much-needed book!" (Rena Lewis, PhD, Professor, College of Education, San Diego State University)*

Humanistic Perspectives on Computers in the Schools, edited by Steven Harlow, PhD (Vol. 1, No. 4, 1985). *"A wide spectrum of information." (Infochange)*

The Web in Higher Education: Assessing the Impact and Fulfilling the Potential has been co-published simultaneously as *Computers in the Schools*™, Volume 17, Numbers 3/4 and Volume 18, Number 1 2001.

First published 2001 by The Haworth Press, Inc.

Published 2020 by Routledge
605 Third Avenue, New York, NY 10017
2 Park Square, Milton Park, Abingdon, Oxon OX14 4RN

Routledge is an imprint of the Taylor & Francis Group, an informa business

ISBN 13: 978-0-7890-1706-2 (hbk)

Cover design by Thomas J. Mayshock Jr.

Library of Congress Cataloging-in-Publication Data

The Web in higher education : assessing the impact and fulfilling the potential / Cleborne D. Maddux, D. LaMont Johnson, editors.
     p. cm.
"Co-published simultaneously as Computers in the schools, volume 17, numbers 3/4 and volume 18, number 1 2001."
Includes bibliographical references and index.
   ISBN 0-7890-1706-7 (hard) – ISBN 0-7890-1707-5 (pbk.)
   1. Internet in higher education. 2. World Wide Web. 3. Educational technology. 4. Information technology. I. Maddux, Cleborne D., 1942- II. Johnson, D. LaMont (Dee LaMont), 1939- III. Computers in the schools.
LB1044.87 .W46 2002
378.1'7344678–dc21

2001133393

The Web
in Higher Education:
Assessing the Impact
and Fulfilling
the Potential

Cleborne D. Maddux
D. LaMont Johnson
Editors

The Web in Higher Education: Assessing the Impact and Fulfilling the Potential has been co-published simultaneously as *Computers in the Schools*, Volume 17, Numbers 3/4 and Volume 18, Number 1 2001.

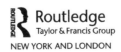

Routledge
Taylor & Francis Group
NEW YORK AND LONDON

Indexing, Abstracting & Website/Internet Coverage

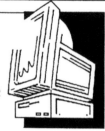

This section provides you with a list of major indexing & abstracting services. That is to say, each service began covering this periodical during the year noted in the right column. Most Websites which are listed below have indicated that they will either post, disseminate, compile, archive, cite or alert their own Website users with research-based content from this work. (This list is as current as the copyright date of this publication.)

(continued)

(continued)

Special Bibliographic Notes related to special journal issues
(separates) and indexing/abstracting:

- indexing/abstracting services in this list will also cover material in any "separate" that is co-published simultaneously with Haworth's special thematic journal issue or DocuSerial. Indexing/abstracting usually covers material at the article/chapter level.
- monographic co-editions are intended for either non-subscribers or libraries which intend to purchase a second copy for their circulating collections.
- monographic co-editions are reported to all jobbers/wholesalers/approval plans. The source journal is listed as the "series" to assist the prevention of duplicate purchasing in the same manner utilized for books-in-series.
- to facilitate user/access services all indexing/abstracting services are encouraged to utilize the co-indexing entry note indicated at the bottom of the first page of each article/chapter/contribution.
- this is intended to assist a library user of any reference tool (whether print, electronic, online, or CD-ROM) to locate the monographic version if the library has purchased this version but not a subscription to the source journal.
- individual articles/chapters in any Haworth publication are also available through the Haworth Document Delivery Service (HDDS).

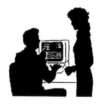

The Web in Higher Education: Assessing the Impact and Fulfilling the Potential

Contents

ABOUT THE EDITORS

Cleborne D. Maddux, PhD, is Professor of Education in the Department of Counseling and Educational Psychology at the University of Nevada, Reno, where he teaches courses on statistics and on integrating technology into education. He trains elementary and high school teachers in the state of Nevada on how to make the Internet a regular feature of their classroom agendas. Senior author of *Educational Computing: Learning with Tomorrow's Technologies,* a textbook now in its third edition, Professor Maddux has authored or co-authored numerous professional articles and books on informational technology in education and educational technology.

D. LaMont Johnson, PhD, is Professor of Education in the Department of Counseling and Educational Psychology at the University of Nevada, Reno. He is also Program Coordinator of the Information Technology in Education program. He teaches courses on the application of technology in education and trains teachers across the state of Nevada in using the Internet in their classrooms. Co-author of the textbook *Educational Computing: Learning with Tomorrow's Technologies,* now in its third edition, Professor Johnson has written or co-written numerous books and articles on educational computing and information technology in education.

Cleborne D. Maddux
D. LaMont Johnson

The Web in Education:
Asset or Liability?

SUMMARY. Computers, the Internet, and the Web are popular educational tools that seem destined to assume even more prominent roles in the future. The question is not whether information technology will survive in schools, but whether or not it will have a revolutionary, or even a positive, effect on teaching and learning. Education in general is facing an array of formidable problems, including sustained and vicious attacks by politicians and business leaders. Possible causes of these attacks are discussed, including generalized anger in the population, the profit motive in the private sector, a belief in "the magic of the marketplace," excessive faith in standardized testing, and growing availability of sophisticated technology for distance education. It remains to be seen whether or not public educators can use information technology to improve traditional, campus-based public education while resisting the pressure to water down their programs for impersonal mass delivery by distance education. *[Article copies available for a fee from The Haworth Document Delivery Service: 1-800-342-9678. E-mail address: <getinfo@haworthpressinc.com> Website: <http://www.HaworthPress.com> © 2001 by The Haworth Press, Inc. All rights reserved.]*

CLEBORNE D. MADDUX is Professor, Department of Counseling and Educational Psychology, University of Nevada, Reno, NV 89557 (E-mail: maddux@unr.edu).
D. LAMONT JOHNSON is Professor, Department of Counseling and Educational Psychology, University of Nevada, Reno, NV 89557.

[Haworth co-indexing entry note]: "The Web in Education: Asset or Liability?" Maddux, Cleborne D., and D. LaMont Johnson. Co-published simultaneously in *Computers in the Schools* (The Haworth Press, Inc.) Vol. 17, No. 3/4, 2001, pp. 1-16; and: *The Web in Higher Education: Assessing the Impact and Fulfilling the Potential* (ed: Cleborne D. Maddux, and D. LaMont Johnson) The Haworth Press, Inc., 2001, pp. 1-16. Single or multiple copies of this article are available for a fee from The Haworth Document Delivery Service [1-800-342-9678, 9:00 a.m. - 5:00 p.m. (EST). E-mail address: getinfo@haworthpressinc.com].

1

KEYWORDS. Distance education, web-enhanced learning, information technology in education

One of the many idiosyncrasies of age may be an increasing proclivity for taking stock of where we have been and for questioning the advisability of where we appear to be going. Since none of us at *Computers in the Schools* is getting any younger, this tendency may be partially responsible for the decision to do a special volume on the Web in Higher Education. In any case, "How We Arrived Here and Where We Seem to Be Going" could serve as an appropriate subtitle.

Reflecting on the developments of the past twenty years reminds us of how incredibly far technology has come in a relatively short period of time. Students in one of my technology classes recently generated a list of technological artifacts that we now consider staples of modern life, but which did not exist less than thirty years ago. That list included, among many others, and in no particular order, *CAT scans, space stations, MRIs, walkmans, camcorders, VCRs, DVDs, CDs, personal computers, laptop computers, handheld computers, fax machines, cordless telephones, cellular telephones, bar codes, laser surgery, automatic teller machines, digital cameras, surround sound, hand-held GPS units, and large-screen television.*

To that impressive list, we would, of course, add the *Internet* and, most fantastic of all, the *World Wide Web*. It almost defies belief to reflect on the fact that there were only about 50 pages on the Web when President Clinton took office. In the last year of the Clinton presidency, there were over *1 billion* Web pages, and growth continues at a breakneck pace!

Looking back at developments in technology as applied to education is only a little less awe-inspiring. In the 1980s and early '90s, I wrote a number of articles expressing my fear that poor implementation might cause the failure of computers in education, and that the first generation of classroom computers might be relegated to the backs of broom closets and storage rooms. Today, I realize that, even if educators made an all-out effort, we could probably not *prevent* the continued increasing presence of computers in classrooms at all levels. Quite simply, in the last five to ten years, computers have gained so much cultural momentum that their continued, growing importance in every walk of life seems assured.

I no longer think that computers in schools are in danger of abandonment. Nevertheless, I must confess that I am not optimistic about the future of education in general, and the role of information technology in particular. Perhaps it is always more comfortable to look to the past than to the future, particularly for those of us who are in the second half (or the fourth quarter) of an educational career.

In any case, it seems to me that the future of public elementary, secondary, and higher education is threatened, at best. We seem to be facing an increasingly formidable array of difficult problems. Of course, there is nothing new about educational problems. Education always has, and probably always will have, its share of difficulties, controversies, and conflicts. However, what seems unprecedented to me is not the number or seriousness of today's problems, but the widespread, often irrational, and frequently *savage* attacks on education that are emanating from many quarters of our society.

It is the sheer *maliciousness* of much of today's spoken and written criticism of education that I find the most startling, and the most discouraging.

I realize that some of this bitter invective is merely a symptom of our times and the evolving American character. Luther Pilkinton (1996), in an editorial for *The Cavalier Daily* at the University of Virginia, characterizes today's Americans as possessing more potential to change their government than do people in any nation in the world, and significantly more even than Americans at any other time in our history. Yet, he asserts, Americans are utterly disillusioned with government, but unwilling to become informed about or positively involved in politics at any level. He concludes that this combination of cynicism and passivity leaves many Americans *angry* (Pilkinton uses a more colorful, but less decorous adjective), *ignorant*, and *powerful*, a dangerous combination that is not consistent with our traditional ideal of participatory government.

Be that as it may, it is *anger* that seems to fuel much modern public commentary in general, and the modern condemnation of education in particular. In fact, it sometimes seems that *rage* has become the defining emotion and the popular avocation, of our times.

Finding support for such a conclusion requires only a brief bit of "dial-surfing" across any of the scores of talk-shows on U.S. radio stations, or a casual scanning of letters to the editor in local newspapers or magazines. In all these forums, hosts, callers, editors, and letter-writers alike seem perpetually *outraged* (and shockingly ill-informed) by the most trivial and obscure as well as the most momentous and popular issues of the day, including a host of educational issues (and, it seems to me, non-issues).

Then, too, anger and indignation are common in many, if not most, of our daily activities. Displays of temper on the highway are so common that a new term–*road rage*–has found its way into the language. The phenomenon is rampant and growing at alarming rates. In fact, a sub-committee of the House Transportation and Infrastructure Committee (1997) reported that since 1990, road rage incidents have increased by 51 percent, resulting in an average of 1,500 fatalities and injuries each year. The previous year, the American Automobile Association (1996) commissioned a study from The Gallup Organization to investigate driver concerns. The study found that 90 percent of surveyed drivers had experienced an incident involving road rage during the previous 12 months, 60 percent admitted to losing their tempers behind the wheel, and a full one percent reported a physical assault by another driver. Furthermore, urban motorists reported feeling more threatened by aggressive drivers than by drunk drivers.

Only this morning, the local newspaper in my community carried a story that coined the term *"cell phone rage."* It seems that people across the country are outraged that some restaurant patrons bring their cell phones to dinner and carry on telephone conversations in the dining room. Those opposed to such cell phone use are voicing complaints to the managers of these establishments, boycotting businesses that refuse to post signs prohibiting cell phone use, and threatening to organize and launch a campaign against the use of cell phones in public places. Some are even confronting cell phone users in restaurants.

The entertainment media routinely exploits anger's popular appeal, making *violence* (the physical manifestation of rage) a staple of prime time television, first-run movies, popular music, and video games. Television programs market hostility and vituperation by featuring "guests" who routinely engage in shrill, profane tirades against each other, and who sometimes carry out physical assaults complete with pushing, punching, and chair-swinging melees. A new media genre, sometimes called *"reality television,"* spotlights interpersonal conflicts and angry recriminations in the daily lives of so-called "ordinary people" in a variety of environments from apartment living rooms to "ship-wreck" islands. Wrestling has become one of the fastest growing "sports" in the country, featuring nearly nonstop, if carefully orchestrated, violence, punctuated with brief periods of hostile, verbal invective.

The media has been (angrily) vilified recently for this penchant for violence. However, it is possible, even likely, that the violence found in mass media offerings is the *effect* rather than the *cause* of a chronically angry and consequently violent society. I suspect that the media moguls are correct (although shamelessly self-serving) when they assert that they merely provide an angry and violent public with the programming they want and with which they can identify.

More uncomfortably close to home, on university campuses across the nation, taking angry offense seems to be the twenty-first century analogue of goldfish swallowing or panty raids. Consequently, academic freedom, once the *sine qua non* of academic life, has given way to political correctness, as university administrators rush to legitimize a generation of students who, like their elders, seem to ache to be offended. Campus after campus has moved to enact policies banning topics or comments that might anger any student or that might be perceived by someone, somewhere, as contributing to a "hostile environment." (Given the current societal and campus penchant for offense, such a policy could probably be used to relegate almost any topic to the forbidden list.) University administrators are continuing these shameful, cowardly, and reactionary regulatory attacks on free speech, despite the fact that in two cases, the United States Supreme Court has overturned speech codes in public universities (Rubin, 1994). One can only hope that Rubin is correct when he opines (in a slightly different context) that, "In a democracy, it is difficult or impossible in the long run to implement policies that lack any intellectual justification."

In a society in which anger and violence are becoming part of the national character, it is not surprising that *courtesy* is falling by the wayside. Many critics have drawn attention to a perceived national decline in *civility*. Perhaps this is an inevitable accompaniment to the escalating ambiance of anger that is sweeping the country. We see a particularly distasteful manifestation at election times, when candidates for offices at all levels appear to compete to outdo each other in sheer nastiness. The entire country witnessed a case in point on the occasion of the nationally televised presidential debates. When candidates for the highest office in the land abandon common courtesy and openly display their contempt for each other, is it surprising that civility is on the wane in the culture at large?

A national epidemic of anger could explain some of the bitter condemnation of education, but is an incomplete explanation at best. Purely irrational, unplanned societal rage, whatever its cause, would likely move randomly from object to object, concentrating its collective ire against first one victim and then another. However, the current tirade against education has continued at a focused and unabated peak since publication of *A Nation at Risk* (1983) nearly twenty years ago.

There are probably many reasons why education has been such a perennial target for so many years. However, one important reason is that the standard bearers of the anti-education movement have consistently been prominent, highly visible individuals from politics and business. These detractors have been relentless in their public condemnation, and they have been spectacularly successful in convincing the public that their criticisms are legitimate.

This brings two questions to mind. First, how have they managed to be so persuasive? Second, what is the motivation for their concentrated, prolonged, and ruthless attack?

Again, there are probably many reasons why the public has been so willing to believe that education in America is hardly worth saving. I have already mentioned the single-minded persistence of its critics over the last twenty years, and the fact that many of these critics are prominent representatives of business and politics. Then, too, many observers have hypothesized that because of events in the '60s and '70s such as political assassinations, Viet Nam and Watergate, Americans have become increasingly willing to believe the worst about any of the activities of their government.

There is probably some truth in that assertion. However, I believe that the increasingly dominant role of anger in the national character (which itself may have been intensified by events in the '60s and '70s) is even more important. It seems to me that the persistent diatribe against education has provided a convenient and familiar focus for the generalized anger of its citizens.

While it is true that anger is directed at many government-related activities, such as those conducted by the Central Intelligence Agency; the Bureau of Alcohol, Tobacco, and Firearms; and the United States Congress; the daily activities of such agencies are largely out of sight and far away from most citizens. Schools, on the other hand, are clearly visible in every neighborhood of every community, and, even more crucially, education deals daily with *children*, whose welfare is more important to most parents than is their own.

Because of these factors, I would judge it remarkable if the educational critics had *not* been highly successful in persuading Americans that their schools are highly deficient. Their success, however, has not been total, as demonstrated by one instructive trend in the results of the annual Gallup poll on the public's attitude toward education. For years, the poll has shown that the majority of parents are at least *satisfied* with their *own* schools, but believe that *other* schools are very poor.

This result is illustrative of the fact that anger is not the only widely shared, American personality trait. Americans have also always had a devotion to fairness in their personal dealings and a willingness to objectively judge the performance of those with whom they are personally acquainted. Thus, while many citizens have been persuaded that schools in general are inferior and teachers are lazy and incompetent, their own experiences with their own schools and teachers are not consistent with this view. Therefore, they conclude that the problems are with other schools and other teachers.

The question of what motivates our political and business leaders to carry on the current crusade against public education is easy to answer, at least with regard to politicians. It is almost axiomatic that politicians need to talk about critical issues. Most voters, if they thought there were no serious and pressing problems to solve, would be even more politically apathetic than they currently are, and would care even less than they currently do about who gets elected. Even more importantly, the media will provide almost unlimited, free publicity to those who claim a crisis exists, particularly a crisis concerning children. This is critical, since no one these days can be elected or reelected without an unhealthy overdose of publicity. Simply put, both politicians and the media are more than willing to exploit the fact that the public, while apathetic about many issues, care deeply about the welfare of their children, and are therefore always willing to listen to anyone who claims they have an educational emergency to reveal and repair, or an educational scandal to expose.

It is more difficult to explain the motivation of business leaders to carry on their current sustained and vitriolic attack on education. This is a much more complex phenomenon, and I suspect there are multiple explanations, including the fact that some people in business are probably genuinely convinced, or at least fearful, that the educational system is as bad as many of their peers have been stridently claiming. After all, people in the business world are as angry as those in other pursuits, and while it seems to be human nature to believe the worst about people and institutions, anger seems to intensify that tendency.

Then, too, there are probably many in business whose condemnation of education stems from their single-minded and sincere belief in what George Soros (1997) has termed "laissez-faire capitalism" (p. 49). Such individuals believe in what Soros terms "the magic of the marketplace" and hold that the private sector is always better than the government at carrying out any activity, and that all such activities should be completely unregulated except by competition.

However, laissez-faire capitalism represents an extreme position, and one not universally endorsed by economists or entrepreneurs. Soros, himself a billionaire entrepreneur, goes further and maintains that laissez-faire capitalism is the dominant belief in our society today, and because communism is no longer the menace it once was, is now a greater global threat than are totalitarian ideologies. Soros argues against laissez-faire capitalism because of its effects on (a) economic stability, (b) social justice, and (c) international relations. As an educator, I am most interested in his comments about social justice. He maintains that all legitimate economic theories assume that people hold firmly established *values* rooted in tradition, religion, and culture. However, a single-minded devotion to market values, he says, undermines traditional values:

> Unsure of what they stand for, people increasingly rely on money as the criterion of value. What is more expensive is considered better. The value of a work of art can be judged by the price it fetches. People deserve respect and admiration because they are rich. What used to be a medium of exchange has usurped the place of fundamental values, reversing the relationship postulated by economic theory. What used to be professions have turned into businesses. The cult of success has replaced belief in principles. Society has lost its anchor. (Soros, 1997, p. 54)

I suspect that many of the entrepreneurs who are harsh critics of education fall into the category of laissez-faire true believers. There are many unfortunate conditions in our society that may result wholly or partly from widespread confidence in this flawed economic theory. Soros does a good job of explaining why the theory is invalid, and identifying some of the larger, cultural outcomes. One of these is the current popularity of a new social Darwinism, by which entrepreneurs rationalize elimination or lack of support for social programs on the evolutionary tenet that only the fit deserve to survive. (This, in spite of the fact that *mutation*, rather than survival of the fittest, is the dominant theme of evolutionary theory, and in any case, *inheritance* of wealth destroys the validity of the analogy.)

The popularity of social Darwinism may explain why many high-tech entrepreneurs do not support charity of any kind. Foster (2000), in a cover story for *Grok*, a high-tech magazine for technology leaders, suggests that technology entrepreneurs, while highly critical of education, have a dismal record of putting their money where their mouths are, whether one considers education or any other social issue:

> Not that the newly wealthy have been tumbling out of the gate when it comes to philanthropy of any kind . . . A survey a few years ago on behalf of Community Foundation Silicon Valley found that one-third of the executives making more than $100,000 per year were donating $1,000 or less to charity. (p. 69)

Another problem with laissez-faire economic theory is that it is an almost unbelievably naïve and simplistic approach to economics and the other affairs of man and government. Faith that completely unrestrained supply and demand will solve all problems is reductionism in the extreme. Additionally, those who subscribe to this approach often tend to see life in general, and education in particular, in similarly naïve and simplistic terms.

Recently, I attended a meeting of educational and community business leaders to discuss educational reform. A millionaire entrepreneur at the meeting stood up to announce proudly that he had the solution for the problems of schools. What educators needed to do, he said, was simply to harness and redirect to academics the enthusiasm children have for baseball and for memorizing baseball statistics. In a later conversation, he was absolutely unwilling to even consider that I might be right when I pointed out that most children in inner city schools (indeed in any schools) do not today share the enthusiasm for memorizing baseball statistics that he had when he was a boy. Even if they did, however, suggesting that this enthusiasm be "redirected to academics" is much easier than doing so.

Granted that the above example may be an extreme, I am always struck by the simplistic approach that business leaders take to educational reform. It is this naivete, I believe, that is responsible for entrepreneurs' single-minded devotion to the concept of standardized testing. Most of the business leaders I have talked with take it for granted that everything worth teaching or learning is measurable with a standardized test. They are utterly closed to the suggestion that the state of the art of testing in education and psychology is in its infancy, and that many of the things we say we value as a people cannot now be measured.

Nor will they credit any suggestion that testing may have undesirable side effects. Instead, they continue to insist that testing is an educational panacea and they advocate increasing the time and money spent in its pursuit. They are completely unmoved by the collective protests of educators such as Vito Perrone (2000), dean of the Harvard Graduate School of Education, who summarized the position of the Association for Childhood Education International (ACEI):

> ACEI strongly believes that no standardized testing should occur in the preschool and K-2 years. Further, ACEI strongly questions the need for testing every child in the remainder of the elementary years. The National Commission on Testing and Public Policy recently reached the same position. The National Association for the Education of Young Children has also called for an end to K-2 testing . . . All testing of young children in preschool and grades K-2 and the practice of testing every child in the later elementary years should cease. To continue such testing in the face of so much evidence of its deleterious effects is the height of irresponsibility.

The insistence on testing in the face of objections by educators and researchers is not an isolated phenomenon. In none of the reform meetings I have attended has there been any attempt to establish an authentic dialogue among politicians, business people, and educators. In fact, it seems to me that the hallmark of the educational reform movement is that many entrepreneurs and politicians are contemptuous of educators, are not at all interested in the opinions of educators, and simply want to tell educators what to do. This would probably not be so difficult for many of us to stomach, if what politicians and business leaders had to say were only a little more workable and realistic, and if their advice did not so often fly in the face of logic and experience.

The suggestion that developing more standardized tests will improve education is one case in point. The Ad Council has produced another in the form of a public service announcement that has been running for months on radio stations across the country. This announcement carries the clear implication that all that really needs to be done to improve education is to give children more difficult work and require them to do it correctly.

This points up one of the characteristics of the reform movement that educators find most unpleasant and insulting–the belief that teaching is essentially easy and educational problems are due to the fact that educators are not really trying to succeed. This cynical view, which ignores the fact that most people in every vocation are hardworking, well-meaning individuals who take pride in their work and do the best they are able, leaves no room for true collaboration or mutual respect, and is counter-productive in every way.

Laissez-faire capitalism is not the only cause for the crusade against education currently being carried out by leaders in business, although capitalism itself is related to yet another motivating factor. I believe that the profit motive itself is responsible for much of the current outcry to scrap public education, establish a voucher system, and empower private schools. Simply put, the business world has begun to recognize that there is money to be made by moving some or all of education out of the public and into the private sector.

It is ironic that much of the current entrepreneurial interest in education has been sparked by the evolution of distance education in general, and the Internet and the World Wide Web in particular. The irony is that while these developments have the potential to revolutionize education in positive ways, they also contain the seeds of destruction of public education, as we know it.

I am not suggesting that there is some national or global conspiracy of entrepreneurs to privatize education. However, I do believe that the potential for profit is contributing, consciously or unconsciously, to the current tendency for business leaders and politicians to denigrate public education and advocate for the educational private sector. Awareness of the potential educational power of the Internet and the Web, the increasing cost-effectiveness of the technology to carry out distance education, and the potential student demand, has suddenly burst upon the business world. Their leaders are licking their entrepreneurial chops in ravenous expectation of the profit-taking gorge to come. Everywhere one turns, they are waxing eloquent about the new opportunities, and making estimates of the profit potential in terms of not millions, but billions of dollars per year.

Many business leaders are making no secret of their aspirations. Ann Krischner, CEO of a company with a Web site financed through a cooperative effort by Columbia University and four other institutions, and dedicated to selling high-prestige courses by distance education, says, without a trace of shame, "We're going to make education a consumer-driven product" (Beiles, 2000).

Estimates certainly don't agree, but last year, we know that online learning companies took in about 500 million dollars, and Merrill Lynch estimates that by 2003, online higher education alone will gross 7 billion dollars a year and continue to grow thereafter at the rate of 55 percent a year (McGinn, 2000). Other estimates run as high as 9 or 10 billion dollars by 2003. In any case, the United States currently spends about 810 billion a year on education, and all indications are that the portion devoted to distance education, both public and private, will continue to increase rapidly. With potential profits like that, is it any wonder that business leaders advocate for the private sector?

More sobering, with potential profits in the billions, is it reasonable to think that business is honestly interested in reforming *public* education? Or is that a little like asking Ford to reform General Motors?

CONCLUSIONS

What is the point of all this? I began with a modest prediction that there are hard times ahead for public education at all levels. The current attacks on education, caused primarily, I believe, by generalized societal anger, political ambition, and entrepreneurial greed, have sparked a host of proposals for "reform."

The current anti-education movement began with publication of the 1983 *Nation at Risk*. That report painted a picture of a nation under siege and at risk from its own educational system. I wonder if our harshest critics ever consider that the "research" for that report is now twenty years old? Those who were in high school at the time are now approaching their 40th birthdays and many are moving into leadership roles in government, business, and industry. Judging by their age, their peers make up the most vigorous portion of the total workforce. If their education was so deficient, how is it that the United States still leads the world in inventions and patents, produces most of the basic science in the world, and has the strongest economy to be found anywhere? How is it that American universities, which now employ a large and rapidly increasing number of professors who were students in our "at risk" educational system in 1983, remain the envy of the rest of the world? In short, if education was so poor in 1980, why are we doing so well in 2000?

The extent of the criticism we now face was illustrated to me recently in a memo from our dean to the faculty of our college. This memo summarized the topics covered in only a few of the meetings he had attended that week. These included *school improvement, stability of staffing, training school leaders, public engagement, parental involvement, funding for educational technology, high-stakes testing, academic standards, class size reduction, differentiated staffing, professional development, teacher mentoring and induction,* and *Title II state report card requirements.* Those reading this article could no doubt easily add substantially to this already imposing list.

The proposals for change implied by many of the topics listed above, because they are largely simplistic and impractical, compound our existing problems, many of which are caused by difficult social conditions in the society at large. This is not to imply that education is without fault, however. Obviously, there is always room for improvement. But improvement, if it comes, is not likely to come from those who suggest we harness and redirect children's enthusiasm for baseball statistics, or through any of the other typically illogical and impractical suggestions that come from politicians and business leaders, many of whom simply want to reinvent the schools of their own youth.

Twenty years ago, I began moving my academic career, which started in special education, into what was a brand new area that we now call *information technology in education.* I did so because I thought I sensed the potential for technology to reenergize and truly reform education by making individualization a practical possibility.

I believe that potential remains viable today. However, sadly, I no longer believe that any degree of educational improvement will satisfy and silence our critics. If I am correct in thinking the criticism stems, not from our performance, but from the factors identified in this article, then improving teaching and learning will have little effect on the rhetoric.

I believe that the Internet and the Web present unique educational opportunities for improving instruction. However, the entrepreneurs seem intent on using the Internet and the Web to privatize and commercialize education. I cannot help but think that totally online courses and programs, whoever creates, markets, and conducts them, are sure to cheapen and weaken education. In higher education, we have all recently witnessed a greatly increased activity level by a host of "diploma mills" which, in effect, sell degrees and offer only a pale shadow of a true academic experience. Some of these commercial institutions make use of the Internet and the Web, and all are planning greatly increased use in the near future.

Some of the patrons of these private diploma mills are merely looking for a "union card" to be used as an entry to a job, and they care not at all about the lack of intellectual challenge or stimulation common to these programs. Faculty are fond of saying, rightly, that we are better off without these individuals. However, other students are there because they are unwilling to tolerate the high-handed manner in which students are traditionally treated on college and university campuses.

Only a brief sampling includes impersonal, rude clerks; long, slow-moving lines; parking permits that are nothing more than expensive permits to search for non-existent spaces; errors in transcripts and grades; and professors who seldom keep appointments or who pride themselves on the numbers of students they are able to fail. To the extent that distance education forces colleges and universities to improve such conditions, they will perform a needed service. However, the changes are unlikely to be that circumscribed.

Among my colleagues, I am known as something of a pessimist, and that assessment is not without some validity. However, I have always maintained that pessimists are nothing more than optimists disillusioned by reality, and I have always endeavored to end my articles in all publications on a hopeful note. For the first time, I find myself hard pressed to do so. I'm not sure I could bring myself to recommend education at any level for my new grandsons. There are simply too many problems and the future is too unsure for a conscionable recommendation.

A few years ago, I would have pointed at the Internet and the Web as one of history's most exciting developments in education. Now, it appears possible that the Internet and the Web will serve only as an instrument to further embattle the already embattled educational enterprise. Schools at all levels, including colleges and universities, seem to be making the critical error of joining, instead of fighting, the commercial diploma mills. Instead of trying to improve what universities traditionally do well in their on-campus programs, while using the Internet and the Web to supplement and improve traditional courses and programs, many campuses are moving to start their own online diploma mills. These public diploma mills will, of course, stand in direct *competition* to their own, on-campus programs.

I can't predict how education will fare in the next ten years. However, I am afraid that things are due to get worse before they get better. The criticism is likely to increase. The dollars are likely to decline. Competition from the private sector is likely to increase. Educational administrators at all levels are likely to continue to pander to politicians and business leaders, especially as public fiscal and moral support continues to decline. The Internet and the Web will continue to increase in importance as a vehicle for public and private course delivery. Rigor and academic respectability are likely to continue to be eroded by totally online offerings.

The open question is whether or not public educators can use information technology to improve traditional, campus-based public education while resisting the pressure to water down their programs for impersonal mass delivery by distance education. It should go without saying that while certain portions of certain courses can be enhanced by employing the Internet and the Web, there are many concepts, topics, and programs that are totally unsuited for delivery by distance education. Einstein is credited with saying "Things should be made as simple as possible–but no simpler."

Perhaps the public needs to be reminded that education and business are incompatible in both means and ends. Business follows the strategy that "the customer is always right," which is believed to lead to profit as the most desirable end. Education, on the other hand, while striving to please as many as possible, must also serve a gate-keeping function. We are charged with withholding credit or a degree from those who do not master the knowledge and skills taught, even though they have paid their tuition. Expertise and mastery, rather than profit, are the ends expected of education. Business, on the other hand, gladly bestows its product on anyone who pays the fee.

The present volume on the Web in Higher Education is partly a product of my own, newly acquired ambivalence about the Web and the role it will play in the future of education. I have been struck by the fact that all the authors of articles in this collection seem convinced that the Web will be a positive force in education. I hope they are right, but I am haunted by the words of Peter Drucker:

> Education will be profoundly changed by the Internet, and higher education most of all. I am not sure that the one American contribution to education, the free-standing four-year college, is going to survive. (Davis, 2000, p. 36)

I am sure it will *not* survive, at least not as we currently know it. The Web is changing virtually every facet of modern life, and it will change education also. I leave it to the authors of articles in this volume, to tell us how they believe education in the 21st century will be transformed by this incredible new technology.

REFERENCES

A Nation at Risk: The Imperative for Educational Reform. (1983). Washington, DC: U.S. Government Printing Office.

American Automobile Association. (1996). Aggressive Driving: Three Studies. Washington, DC: AAA Foundation for Traffic Safety. Retrieved October 5, 2000, from the World Wide Web: *http://www.aaafts.org/Text/research/agdrtext.htm#Road Rage*

Beiles, N. (2000, October). A league of her own. *Grok*, pp. 40-44.

Davis, J. (2000, October). Class acts. *Grok*, pp. 27-36.

Foster, D. (2000, October). Paying the price. *Grok*, pp. 66-74.

House Transportation and Infrastructure Committee. (1997). Road rage: Causes and dangers of aggressive driving. Washington, DC: Author. Retrieved October 5, 2000, from the World Wide Web: *http://www.house.gov/transportation/surface/sthearin/ist717/ist717.htm*

McGinn, D. (2000, October). Biz men on campus. *Grok*, pp. 76-84.

Perrone, V. (2000) On standardized testing. Retrieved October 6, 2000, from the World Wide Web: *http://ericps.ed.uiuc.edu/eece/pubs/digests/1991/perron91.html*

Pilkinton, L. B. (1996, April 18). Pissed off, ignorant, powerful. *The Cavalier Daily*. Charlottesville, VA: The University of Virginia.

Rubin, P. (1994). The assault on the First Amendment: Public choice and political correctness. *The CATA Journal, 14*(1). Retrieved October 5, 2000, from the World Wide Web: *http://www.cato.org/pubs/journal/cj14n1-3.html*

Soros, G. (1997). The capitalist threat. *The Atlantic Monthly, 279*(2), pp. 45-58.

Carol B. MacKnight

Supporting Critical Thinking
in Interactive Learning Environments

SUMMARY. The aim of this paper is to investigate the utilization of critical thinking in different applications and in different types of learning environments. The art of analytical reading includes the same skills as those involved in the art of problem solving and communicating. These skills are essential to the process of filtering, assimilating, and finding new meaning in the torrents of information faced daily. Described are a problem-solving environment and Web communication systems, with the suggestion that the Web tools have not yet come up to faculty expectations for teaching and learning. *[Article copies available for a fee from The Haworth Document Delivery Service: 1-800-342-9678. E-mail address: <getinfo@haworthpressinc.com> Website: <http://www.HaworthPress.com> © 2001 by The Haworth Press, Inc. All rights reserved.]*

KEYWORDS. Critical thinking online, reading critically, critical questioning, analytical skills, knowledge creation, problem solving, inquiry-based learning

The intellectual gap between those who enter college able to read critically and those who have difficulty even in identifying an author's major thesis may be the single most important issue in postsecondary education (Orndorff, 1987). Reading is an active, thinking process

CAROL B. MACKNIGHT is Instructional Technologist, Office of Information Technologies, Lederle Graduate Research Center, University of Massachusetts, Amherst, MA 01003 (E-mail: cmacknight@oit.umass.edu).

[Haworth co-indexing entry note]: "Supporting Critical Thinking in Interactive Learning Environments." MacKnight, Carol B. Co-published simultaneously in *Computers in the Schools* (The Haworth Press, Inc.) Vol. 17, No. 3/4, 2001, pp. 17-32; and: *The Web in Higher Education: Assessing the Impact and Fulfilling the Potential* (ed: Cleborne D. Maddux, and D. LaMont Johnson) The Haworth Press, Inc., 2001, pp. 17-32. Single or multiple copies of this article are available for a fee from The Haworth Document Delivery Service [1-800-342-9678, 9:00 a.m. - 5:00 p.m. (EST). E-mail address: getinfo@haworthpressinc.com].

(Adler & Van Doren, 1972; Spiro, 1980). It helps students construct meaning from a book or a research article, participate in online course discussion, and evaluate resources on the Web. Orndorff (1987) suggests that students' inability to read critically is related to the fact that this skill has not been widely taught.

Students are introduced to elementary reading, making sense of words and sentences, in the early years of their schooling. By junior high, some students may be able to complete what Adler and Van Doren (1972) call an inspectional reading; that is, they can answer what the book is about, what its structure and parts are, and identify the kind of book it is. Students, however, continue to have trouble with these first two levels of reading. Few, upon entering college, progress to the third level of reading, analytical reading, where the reader asks many organized, critical questions of what is read. Still fewer are capable of reading many books on a topic and able to construct an analysis that may not be in any of them, in effect, create new knowledge (Adler & Van Doren, 1972; Browne & Keeley, 1986; Jonassen, 1996).

Following is an examination of the essence of active reading, a kind of "talking back" to the author, and a description of how the art and skill involved in interacting with texts are utilized in a problem-solving environment on the Web and possibly underutilized in online communication tools. It is argued that analytical skills must be taught and that the Web could offer an appropriate environment for developing and using insightful reading skills.

WHAT IS READING REALLY?

Some students are naturally gifted interrogators of information and capable of evaluating a wide variety of resources. Many others have to learn how to interact with texts. To get the most out of a journal article, critique of a book or a poem, the active reader must engage in a critical-questioning strategy. It is not enough to simply get the overall idea of what the book is about, an inspectional reading. This is a necessary step, but it represents a more passive approach, a reading purely for information or entertainment, than the one required to develop critical thinking for analytical reading described below.

Being a Demanding Reader

The techniques that reviewers and editors apply to books and articles are those that active readers also employ when interacting with the author and the text. They read a book, as they would look at a house with an orderly arrangement of rooms. Each room may be an independent unit but, nevertheless, relate in such a way to the other spaces as to make the whole useful, and the architectural plan intelligible. Reviewers, like all good readers, find the author's organizational plan by asking appropriate questions.

Indeed, "None of the more complex steps in the critical-reading process is particularly helpful until the [pattern of] organization is discovered" (Browne & Keeley, 1986, p. 9). What is the structure? What are the parts? What are the major organizational functions that sentences and paragraphs offer that good readers look for as they read? The important parts of the structure are the leading theme and the arguments–issues, reasons, and conclusion(s). The critical question to ask of each is "what?" followed by "why?"

Critical reading is a sorting-out process. Active readers search for the writer's reasoning, which may not always be obvious. They question whether important elements are present, whether those present are clear, and chafe at those elements in an article that don't belong there. They are active searchers in a dialog with the writer, asking critical questions, as all good readers should do.

Acquiring "question-asking" skills begin with knowing the right questions to ask and applying them to a variety of reading materials, from a research article to a novel. In their book, *Asking the Right Questions*, Browne and Keeley list the following questions as a precondition for critical thinking:

1. What are the issue[s] and the conclusion[s]?
2. What are the reasons?
3. What words or phrases are ambiguous?
4. What are the value conflicts and assumptions?
5. What are the definitional and descriptive assumptions?
6. Are the samples representative and the measurements valid?
7. Are there flaws in the statistical reasoning?
8. Are there alternative causal explanations?
9. Are there any errors in reasoning?
10. What significant information is omitted?
11. What alternative conclusions are consistent with the strong reasons?
12. What are your value preferences in this controversy? (Brown & Keeley, 1986, p. 8).

Active readers use their analytical skills preeminently for the sake of understanding. They are not the type of readers who finish a book only to start another, and who may, therefore, become superficially acquainted with a large number of books (Adler & Van Doren, 1972). Good readers not only evaluate the significance of what they are reading, but also spend time in reflection (Harste, 1986). The seeds of ideas that emerge from their reflections are often discussed in classrooms, book clubs, and coffee shops. And sometimes, after refining these ideas, these seeds grow beyond the condition of personal understanding and become new knowledge for others to use.

Traditionally, books have been an important tool in our endeavors to move from understanding less to understanding more. "If we want to go on learning, then we must know how to learn from books" (Adler & Van Doren, 1972, p. 115). It is an impossible task to learn more from books without at least some skill in analytical reading: being able to define the problem or problems that the author is trying to resolve (Adler & Van Doren, 1972). To go on reading actively requires not only the willingness, but also the skills to do so. Like all skills, acquiring them takes practice. Analytical skills are not reserved only for reading, for all forms of communication require them. They can, therefore, be transferred to diverse applications, as we will see later in this article.

The creation of new knowledge rests on students' well-developed capabilities to problem solve and think critically.[1] Those who excel are those who can go beyond collecting information and can add new value to information. "Faced with the explosion of information and its fragmentation, . . . the faculties of our universities are confronted with the difficult choice of balancing analysis with synthesis, methodology, and the relevant course content, thus placing more and more responsibility on the student to form his own syntheses" (Gregorian, 1996, p. 599). New technologies give us the tools and resources to help students develop critical-thinking skills and establish coherence, connection, and meaning in many disciplines.

In the next section, an online problem-solving environment is described, the Knowledge Integration Environment,[2] which focuses on the development of similar skills to those used in analytical reading. The Knowledge Integration Environment uses Web-based tools developed specifically to structure learning activities in science that address student misconceptions, and that seek student elaboration of their answers and justification of their responses through discussion, interactive questioning, and group presentations.

MAKING THE PROBLEM-SOLVING PROCESS VISIBLE

The Knowledge Integration Environment[3] is a joint project between higher education (engineering and education) and public schools. It offers a learning environment that "uses the Internet to help middle and high school students develop an integrated understanding of science and a critical eye toward the complex resources found on the Web" (Knowledge Integration Environment, 1997, p. 1).

The Knowledge Integration Environment is based on Scaffolded Knowledge Integration, a framework developed through more than 10 years of cognitive research on students' scientific thinking and influenced by Vygotsky's work on social interaction in cooperative learning and scaffolding. Scaffolding is the process of providing the help and guidance necessary for solving problems that are slightly more difficult than those that students can tackle independently (Collins, Brown, & Newman, 1989; Palincsar & Brown, 1984).

The Knowledge Integration Environment students begin their project by stating their own opinion about a scientific question or theory, such as heat transfer. Will aluminum foil or wool keep something hot that has been taken out of the oven? Students restate the problem identifying what they already know about it, and what they need to learn. Then they search the Internet for evidence; evaluate the quality of evidence; create evidence through observations, experiments, and simulations; organize evidence; develop an argument; and conclude with a classroom debate, in which students present their arguments and supporting evidence, and field questions from the rest of the class. There are many similarities in this process to those used by a critical reader who continually asks questions of the author, reflects on these questions, and discusses points of understanding, disagreement, or confusion with others.

A key feature of the Knowledge Integration Environment is its suite of online tools for problem solving (see Table 1). These tools help students "express and reflect on their conceptual ideas about scientific phenomena, explore and compare their ideas to those of others, and make sound discriminations between the set of models under consideration" (Bell, 1997, p. 2).

Supporting Group Argumentation and Knowledge Construction

The SenseMaker tool in the Knowledge Integration Environment "provides a spatial and categorical representation for a collection of Web-based evidence" (Bell, 1997, p. 2). It allows groups of students to

TABLE 1. Online Tools for the Knowledge Integration Environment

Tools	Function
Checklist	Tracks what they have done; what is left to be done; and how to do it
Mildred the Cow	Serves as an online guide providing cognitive guidance
Note Taking	A place to write ideas and evidence down
SenseMaker	Allows students to organize evidence into a coherent scientific argument
Evidence Database	A collection of individual pieces of evidence
SpeakEasy	Allows students to exchange and evaluate scientific ideas with classmates, other students, and scientists over the Internet

organize, annotate, and rate a collection of evidence associated with their project. As part of the process, students use the online Guide component to elaborate on their scientific ideas and SenseMaker to develop broad conceptual categories in which to group the evidence. SenseMaker has built-in scaffolding to help students as they create new frames (categories) for their evidence. It also has a Frame Library, modeling good examples and criteria for new conceptual categories. Research indicates "SenseMaker arguments can foster meaningful collaboration between students by making thinking visible between the individuals involved" (Bell, 1997, p. 7).

To add to our knowledge, it is helpful to test and solidify new ideas with others. Oral communication–student-student, student-teacher, student-class–is also an important component of the Knowledge Integration Environment. The Knowledge Integration Environment succeeds, says Marcia Linn, a professor at the University of California at Berkeley, "by helping students link, connect, distinguish, compare, and analyze their repertoire of ideas" (Linn, 1996, April, p. 34).

The Knowledge Integration Environment offers an exciting online environment for students and teachers in their exploration of scientific ideas. Its integrated suite of tools helps learners establish a visual picture of the complex process involved in problem solving and decisionmaking. The built-in tools support them in their investigations in an inquiry-based pedagogy and help them become improved problem solvers. The Checklist, a form of labeling, tracks what needs to be done next, helping the teacher maintain the role of facilitator and giving students more self-directed responsibility for their own learning and knowledge creation.

Most importantly, students gain lifelong learning skills relating to the use of evidence in supporting arguments and the interpretation of current scientific debates, such as the deformed frog controversy. Collected evidence is evaluated and color-coded according to its importance in supporting the competing hypotheses–a chemical hypothesis or a parasite hypothesis–that explain the cause of the current deformity found in frogs.

In the final section, the potential of online communication tools (e-mail, distribution lists, bulletin boards, group forums, and conferences) is considered as it applies to advancing critical thinking, and building collaborative communities of learners.

CAN WEB COMMUNICATION TOOLS
PROMOTE CRITICAL THINKING?

The potential of the Web for establishing communication and collaboration among individuals and groups has long been recognized as one of its major features. Faculty has used the Web to conduct group discussions that could not be effectively handled in class due to time constraints and class size. The quality of the discussions, however, has been mixed. In those cases where quality was relatively poor, major reasons given were unclear objectives and requirements, insufficient mentoring, and lack of critical-thinking skills. With respect to the performance of students in discussing a text just read, the National Assessment of Educational Progress (1981) noted:

> Students seem satisfied with their initial interpretations of what they have read and seem genuinely puzzled at a request to explain or defend their point of view. As a result, responses to assessment items requiring explanations of criteria, analysis of texts or defense of a judgmental point of view were disappointing. Few students could provide more than superficial responses to such tasks, and even the "better" responses showed little evidence of well developed problem-solving or critical thinking skills. (pp. 28-29)

Online communications put emphasis on student comprehension and knowledge of the elements of an argument. We cannot assume that all students will come with sufficient critical thinking skills to advance an online conversation. The building blocks of an argument must become second nature to students. If we want to get beyond the point of "I agree with Harry's statement," then we must consider the issues described earlier that focus on the process of reading critically for understanding. Throughout their educational studies, students should have repeated opportunities to practice critical thinking.

Techniques for Monitoring Discussions

In current communication tools on the Web, the instructor must demonstrate the quality of critical thinking. Acting as a coach or facilitator, the instructor models critical thinking with Socratic questions that are designed to clarify, summarize, probe, and move the students' thinking along (Paul, 1996). Exactly what is to be achieved from thinking critically is stated by the National Council for Excellence in Critical Thinking:

> Disciplined thinking with respect to any subject involves the capacity on the part of the thinker to recognize, analyze, and assess the basic elements of thought: the purpose or goal of thinking; the problem or question at issue; the frame of reference or points of view involved; assumptions made; central concepts and ideas at work; principles or theories used; evidence, data, or reasons advanced; claims made and conclusions drawn; inferences, reasoning, and lines of formulated thought; and implications and consequences involved. (National Council for Excellence in Critical Thinking, p. 1)

Online communication tools do not address the elements of critical thinking described in this paper. Therefore, questions raised by the instructor, acting as a facilitator, become critical and the role of the facilitator more demanding. A few examples of Socratic questioning reported here are taken from Paul and Binker (1990) and may serve as one line of questioning students who are participating in bulletin boards, conferencing (a system for enabling written, online group discussions), or e-mail (see Figure 1).

Effective Communications

As participants in online discussions, students should ask themselves several questions. The first question is what makes a good conversation or discussion? Bronson Alcott, an innovative educator in the nineteenth century, thought conversation to be the most important school activity (MacKnight, 1996). His conversational method has been described in these terms:

FIGURE 1. Questions for Online Facilitators

Socratic Questioning

Questions for Clarification

13. What do you mean by_____?
• What is your main point?
• Could you give me an example?
• What do you think the main issue is here?

Questions that Probe Assumptions
• What are you assuming?
• What could we assume instead?
• How would you justify taking this for granted?
• Is this always the case?

Questions that Probe Reasons and Evidence
• What would be an example?
• Could you explain your reasons to us?
• Are those reasons adequate?
• Do you have any evidence for that?

Questions about Viewpoints or Perspectives
• How would other groups of people respond? Why?
• How could you answer the objection that ____would make?
• Can anyone see this another way?
• What would someone who disagrees say?

Questions that Probe Implications and Consequences
• What are you implying by that?
• What effect would that have?
• What is an alternative?
• If this is the case, then what else must be true?

Questions About the Initial Question or Issue
• How can we find out?
• Can we break this question down at all?
• What does this question assume?
• Why is this question important?

(From Font, Todd, & Welch, 1996, p. 4)

Conversation was no mere question-and-answer session for Alcott. It was a mood, an atmosphere; it was a work of art as surely as were paintings or symphonies. Alcott especially liked the analogy to a symphony. He believed that the ideal conversation developed a single theme and presented it in a variety of ways, providing the greatest scope and freedom for the genius of the participants. Each of the participants would contribute his or her ideas about the theme, thus presenting differing expressions of the theme like the various instruments in an orchestra. All would blend together in beautiful harmony as the session progressed. (Dahlstrand, 1945, p. 216)

This definition of a conversation constitutes a well-developed argument: Conversation is an art (claim); participants presented differing perspectives (evidence); all came to a shared meaning on the issue (conclusion). The aim of education, Alcott declared, is "the production and original exercise of thought [not the learning of facts and the production of right or wrong answers]" (McCuskey, 1940, p. 32).

Face-to-face conversations or discussions differ from online discussion in several respects. In a classroom setting, the instructor can immediately refocus or redirect the conversation. Feedback can also be quickly provided, but given to fewer students in most classroom settings. Online, asynchronous conversation may allow for increased participation, greater reflection, giving and accepting feedback, group process skills, and achieving negotiation skills. It is important, then, for online participants to be aware of the significance of their responses. In developing the critical thinking skills, it is necessary to help students assess textual materials in light of the following questions.

1. What is the goal of the activity?
2. How will my contribution advance the conversation?
3. How would I evaluate my contribution?
4. Are there errors in my reasoning?
5. How good is my evidence?
6. Are there alternative causal explanations?
7. What significant information is omitted?
8. How close are we to solving the problem?

Getting students to think critically over a networked environment can be time consuming for the facilitator, states Goddard (1996), particularly when the class size is larger than 15 students. Chong (1998) affirms the difficulties of managing asynchronous discussions and enumerates some of the management challenges facilitators must consider that arise in large classes. To meet the many challenges, faculty must be prepared to make some changes such as:

1. Increasing their preparation time for successful online activities
2. Blocking off sufficient training time for both instructors and students

3. Giving timely and appropriate feedback to large numbers of students
4. Assessing student progress when the amount of data can be unmanageable
5. Reviewing task clarity and expectations frequently
6. Providing support strategies and personnel for technical and course assistance
7. Establishing clear grading criteria when assessment models may not exist

Chong writes that the amount of information presented in an online conference is often overwhelming to students.

Instructionally Relevant Communication Tools

Unlike the Knowledge Integration Environment's problem-solving environment, many online communication tools (bulletin boards, conferences, forums, etc.) fail to meet the immediate instructional needs of faculty who are engaged in critical inquiry. By their lack of structure, these tools imply that discussions are just "talk." However, for many students, interacting with content effectively and interacting socially to construct meaning are skills that need to be developed. Bulletin boards, conferences, and forums proliferate with examples of students responding to statements or questions by talking past each other, possibly with a grade in mind. This often happens when the task and expectations are unclear to students and peer interaction isn't appreciated or is seen as criticism. Students need to be able to construct their own knowledge: reformulating it, making it their own personal interpretation, sharing it with others, and building on these ideas through the reaction and responses of peers (Brown & Thompson, 1997). They must understand the elements of critical thinking and exercise this thinking. Faculty, on the other hand, must possess the requisite skills necessary to help students become conscious of their process of inquiry. Their job as a facilitator is made that much harder because of the lack of sophistication of current communication tools.

The communication tools found on the Web were not designed with pedagogical goals in mind. They were designed to attract a general audience with their ease of use. The options for participation are often restricted to the posting of comments and responses in a single format. The process of accessing comments by individual students in a threaded discussion is often unwieldy. Vaughn (1999), in addressing some of the limitations of

WebCT bulletin boards, speaks of a need to limit the number of messages displayed while still providing a way for students to know what they have and have not read. To meet some basic faculty requirements, homegrown communication tools have appeared on individual campuses. These tools organize messages by topic, and by student, and by time, and send student responses directly into the student's portfolio for easy access in grading. But, these improvements only offer better course management support. They, too, lack the pedagogical supports mentioned below.

What remains inadequate in Web communication tools are features that support critical thinking and group processes, and that enhance the facilitator's ability to offer constructive guidance on problem solving and critical thinking. For distance education, tools that provide appropriate structure for different communication needs–brainstorming, defining problems, generating questions, analyzing evidence, drawing conclusions or solutions–are essential (Duffy, Dueber, & Hawley, 1998). Bonk and Dennen (1999) further suggest that activities that support critical thinking (structured debates, case analysis, rebuttals, etc.) might be made available to learners in an environment containing templates for critical-thinking activities. Without some built-in structure for solving problems or other supports in Web tools (such as those demonstrated by the Knowledge Integration Environment) that develop students' mental faculties in critical thinking, students may be at a loss whenever critical considerations are required. Until educators and developers work together toward developing pedagogically sound communication tools, the missing piece in online courses will continue to be a "natural" collaborative system that allows groups the means to define what they know, question what they believe, identify weak arguments, and foster new discoveries (Keeley, 1997).

CONCLUSION

Reading books need not be a reclusive experience between the reader and author. Once readers know the right questions to ask of the author and reflect on the material, they can discuss their understanding with others on the Web and build conceptual connections to their own knowledge base. The Web, through its community of users, provides unlimited human resources with whom readers can share their knowledge. The American Literature site (http://www.cwrl.utexas.edu/~daniel/amlit/survey.html) is a good example. When students posted their analyses of books read in an American literature class, they received interactive comments from all over the United States. In fact, when the course ended, students continued to receive comments on their interpretations of the author's use of certain literary techniques.

The Knowledge Integration Environment is a wonderful example of providing a strong online support system to help students arrive at a personal understanding of science by utilizing a problem-solving environment. It offers another avenue for developing critical thinking skills. Many students will not major in science, says Marcia Linn (1996), but we do need to help students know enough about science that they can become critics of information and be capable of critiquing evidence in various media formats, including films, photographs, and persuasive speeches in order to perform their civic duties: to vote, to serve on juries, to preserve the environment, etc.–to act as knowledgeable human beings.

Finally, as Paul states, "critical thinking is not a separate set of skills separable from excellence in communication, problem-solving, creative thinking, or collaborative learning" (Willsen & Binker, 1993, p. 93). The analysis of texts, or the thought process applied in a problem-solving situation, uses the same skills that are needed in the creation of new knowledge. Critical thinking skills–the ability to reorganize knowledge in meaningful and usable ways–are essential to the creation of new knowledge.

How well current Web communication tools meet the needs of an intellectually diverse body of students is debatable. By themselves, the available Web tools do not provide aids for the development of critical thinking. The expectation in using them is that students and facilitators will already possess critical thinking skills–assessing information, analyzing ideas and their organization, and connecting relationships between objects or events and theories. However, their potential can be extended through better-designed tools for self-learners, distance learners, and others as they pursue inquiry-based learning and practice using critical thinking skills. These tools can be designed to teach thinking skills and help users work out solutions to problems, illustrating important ideas about thinking and problem solving as it is going on.

Customizing a Web space into a critical-learning environment with embedded supports to facilitate knowledge building and socio-affective activities is a highly desirable endeavor. Students will need experience in interacting with a variety of different information resources and tools and will need opportunities to sharpen their skills in inquiry-based learning, individually and in collaboration with others. In this century, students will live in a networked, global society where knowledge may very well be the most critical resource for future economic development (Harasim, 1995). We must prepare them.

NOTES

1. Critical thinking includes the ability to respond to material by distinguishing between facts and opinions or personal feelings, judgments and inferences, inductive and deductive arguments, and the objective and subjective. It also includes the ability to generate questions, construct and recognize the structure of arguments, and adequately support arguments; define, analyze, and devise solutions for problems and issues; sort, organize, classify, correlate, and analyze materials and data; integrate information and see relationship; evaluate information, materials, and data by drawing inferences, arriving at reasonable and informed conclusions, applying understanding and knowledge to new and different problems, developing rational and reasonable interpretations, suspending beliefs by assimilating information and remaining open to new information, methods, cultural systems, values and beliefs. (MCC General Education Initiatives, p. 2, *http://www.kcmetro.cc.mo.us/longview/ctac/definitions.htm*)

2. Other systems worthy of learning more about are the Computer-Supported Intentional Learning Environment (CSILE) and the Collaborative Visualization project (CoVis). CSILE has been used in many disciplines with primary and secondary students. In a CSILE classroom students are required to label their contributions: What I need to know; What I need to understand; high-level questions, new learning, plan, my theory, new experiment, conclusion, and synthesis (Oshima, 1994); "The labels serve to mentor students in the elements of inquiry in a way analogous to the facilitator in a problem-based learning environment. That is, students must think about how their entry contributes to the problem-solving effort" (Duffy, Dueber, & Hawley, 1999, p. 62). Both CSILE and CoVIS address pedagogical goals. CoVIS, developed at Northwestern University, has similar functions to those of CSILE. High school students, for example, use the Notebook for collaborative inquiry about science problems. Here, too, students must label how their entry contributes to the inquiry: information, commentary, question, conjecture, evidence for, evidence against, plan, and step in plan (Duffy, Dueber, & Hawley, 1999; Edelson & O'Neill, 1994).

3. The Knowledge Integration Environment (KIE) has a change of name, the Web-based Integrated Science Environment (WISE). In this paper I refer to the original in terms of goals, which remain the same, and to WISE in the description of the latest tools. Both are available at:

KIE: *http://www.kie.berkeley.edu/KIE/curriculum/curriculum.html*
WISE: *http://wise.berkeley.edu/WISE/pages/about.html*

REFERENCES

Adler, M.J., & Van Doren, C. (1972). *How to read a book*. New York: Simon & Schuster.

Bell, P. (1997). Using argument representations to make thinking visible for individuals and groups. In R. Hall, N. Miyake, & N. Enyedy (Eds.), *Proceedings of CSCL '97: The Second International Conference on Computer Support for Collaborative Learning* (pp. 10-19). Toronto: University of Toronto Press.

Bonk, C.J., & Dennen, V. (1999). Teaching on the Web: With a little help from my pedagogical friends. *Journal of Computing in Higher Education, 11*(1), 3-29.

Brown, A., & Thompson, H. (1997). *Course design for the WWW: Keeping online students onside* [Online]. Available: *http://www.curtin.edu.au/conference/ascilite97/papers/Brown/Brown.html* [1999, August 20].

Browne, M.N., & Keeley, S.M. (1986). *Asking the right questions.* Englewood Cliffs, NJ: Prentice-Hall.

Chong, S.M. (1998). Models of asynchronous computer conferencing for collaborative learning in large college classes. In C.J. Bonk & K.S. King (Eds.), *Electronic collaborators* (pp. 157-182). Mahwah, NJ: Lawrence Erlbaum.

Collins, A., Brown, J.S., & Newman, S.E. (1989). Cognitive apprenticeship: Teaching the crafts of reading, writing, and mathematics. In L.B. Resnick (Ed.), *Knowing, learning, and instruction: Essays in honor of Robert Glaser* (pp. 453-494). Hillsdale, NJ: Lawrence Erlbaum.

Dahlstrand, F.C. (1945). *Amos Bronson Alcott.* London and Toronto: Associated University Presses.

Duffy, T.M., Dueber, B., & Hawley, C.L. (1998). Critical thinking in a distributed environment: A pedagogical base for the design of conferencing systems. In C.J. Bonk & K.S. King (Eds.), *Electronic collaborators: Learner-centered technologies for literacy, apprenticeship, and discourse* (pp. 51-78). Mahwah, NJ: Lawrence Erlbaum.

Edelson, D.C., & O'Neill, D.K. (1994, April). *The CoVis collaboratory notebook: Computer support for scientific inquiry.* Paper presented at the annual meeting of the American Educational Research Association, New Orleans.

Font, M., Todd, G., & Welch, B. (1996). *What is critical thinking?* [Online] Available: *http://www.iusb.edu/~msherida/tctstud.html* [1999, August 20].

Goddard, J.M. (1996). E for engagement, E for e-mail. *Proceedings of ASCILITE '96 Conference.* Adelaide, Australia, 13, 211-220.

Gregorian, V. (1996). Technology, scholarship, and the humanities: The implications of electronic information. In R. Kling (Ed.), *Computerization and controversy* (pp. 597-605). San Diego, CA: Academic Press.

Harasim, L.M. (1995). *Interacting in hyperspace* [Online]. Available: *http://www.umuc.edu/ide/potentialweb97/harasim.html* [1999, September 3].

Harste, J.C. (1986, December 2-6). *What it means to be strategic: Good readers as informants.* Paper presented at the 36th Annual Meeting of the National Reading Conference, Austin, TX. (ERIC Document Reproduction Service No. ED 278 980)

Jonassen, D.H. (1996). *Computers in the classroom: Mindtools for critical thinking.* Englewood Cliffs, NJ: Prentice Hall.

Keeley, L. (1997, Nov/Dec). Designing for an educational revolution. *Educom Review,* pp. 12-14.

Knowledge Integration Environment. (1997). [Online]. Available: *http://www.kie.berkeley.edu/KIE/tour/KIEtour.html* [1999, August 20].

Linn, M. (1996, April). Key to the information highway. *Communications of the ACM, 39*(4), 34-35.

Linn, M. (1996). *Keynote speaker.* National Council for Excellence in Critical Thinking. Boston: ED-MEDIA. [Online]. Available: *http://www.criticalthinking.org/ncect.nck* [1999, August 20].

MacKnight, C.B. (1996, December 2-4). Changing educational paradigms (Keynote Address). *Proceedings of ASCILITE '96 Conference, 13* (pp. 15-33). Adelaide, Australia.

McCuskey, D. (1940). *Bronson Alcott, teacher.* New York: Macmillan.

National Assessment of Educational Progress publications (1981). Denver, CO: Education Commission of the States.

National Council for Excellence in Critical Thinking (1996). [Online] Available: *http://www.criticalthinking.org/ncect.nclk* [1999, August 20].

Orndorff, J. (1987, April 9-12). *Using computers and original text to teach critical reading and thinking.* Paper presented at the Meeting of the Conference on Critical Thinking. Newport News, VA.

Oshima, J. (1994, April). *Coordination of solo- and joint-plan of student activity in CSILE: Analysis from the perspective of activity theory by Leontiev and Engestrom.* Paper presented at the annual meeting of the American Educational Research Association, New Orleans.

Palincsar, A.S., & Brown, A. L. (1984). Reciprocal teaching of comprehension-fostering and monitoring activities. *Cognition and Instruction, 1,* 117-175.

Paul, R. (1996). *How to teach through Socratic questioning.* Transcript of a three-part video series. Santa Rosa, CA: Foundation for Critical Thinking.

Scardamalia, M., & Bereiter, C. (1996). Adaptation and understanding: A case for new cultures of schooling. In S. Vosniado, E. DeCorte, R. Glaser, & H. Mandl (Eds.), *International perspectives on the design of technology-supported learning environments* (pp. 149-163). Mahwah, NJ: Lawrence Erlbaum.

Spiro, R.J. (1980). Constructive processes in prose comprehension and recall. In R.J. Spiro (Ed.), *Theoretical issues in reading comprehension* (pp. 245-278). Hillsdale, NJ: Lawrence Erlbaum.

Vaughn, M. (1999, May). *Article No. 354.* Response in a private forum on WebCT Bulletin Board for Users.

Willsen, J., & Binker, A.J.A. (Eds.). (1993). *Critical thinking.* Santa Rosa, CA: Foundation for Critical Thinking.

Pamela T. Northrup
Karen Rasmussen

Considerations for Designing Web-Based Programs

SUMMARY. With over two million students projected to be enrolled in higher education distance learning courses by the year 2002, it is imperative that consideration be given to the design of high-quality online programs. Using the framework of grounded design as a context for dealing with the range of design decisions that best facilitate learning outcomes, five areas are discussed: psychological, pedagogical, technical, cultural, and pragmatic (Hannafin, Hannafin, Land, & Oliver, 1997). Examples are provided of how each area of grounded design can be used, as instructional designers, content experts, and others establish Web-based programs in higher education. *[Article copies available for a fee from The Haworth Document Delivery Service: 1-800-342-9678. E-mail address: <getinfo@haworthpressinc.com> Website: <http://www.HaworthPress.com> © 2001 by The Haworth Press, Inc. All rights reserved.]*

KEYWORDS. Web-based programs, graduate degrees, grounded theory, constructivism, instructional design, learning outcomes, distance education, online learning, online programs, student-centered, instructional technology

PAMELA T. NORTHRUP is Director, Educational Research and Development Center, Division of Technology, Research and Development, University of West Florida, 11000 University Parkway, Pensacola, FL 32514 (E-mail: pnorthru@uwf.edu).
KAREN RASMUSSEN is Coordinator of Instructional Technology and Associate Professor, Division of Technology, Research, and Development, University of West Florida, 11000 University Parkway, Pensacola, FL 32514 (E-mail: krasmuss@uwf.edu).

[Haworth co-indexing entry note]: "Considerations for Designing Web-Based Programs." Northrup, Pamela T., and Karen Rasmussen. Co-published simultaneously in *Computers in the Schools* (The Haworth Press, Inc.) Vol. 17, No. 3/4, 2001, pp. 33-46; and: *The Web in Higher Education: Assessing the Impact and Fulfilling the Potential* (ed: Cleborne D. Maddux, and D. LaMont Johnson) The Haworth Press, Inc., 2001, pp. 33-46. Single or multiple copies of this article are available for a fee from The Haworth Document Delivery Service [1-800-342-9678, 9:00 a.m. - 5:00 p.m. (EST). E-mail address: getinfo@haworthpressinc.com].

INTRODUCTION

By 2002, over two million college students will be enrolled in distance learning courses. It is anticipated that higher education institutions will develop distance learning programs in an attempt to meet the demand, with approximately 84% of four-year colleges and universities participating (Council for Higher Education Accreditation, 2000).

With this tremendous growth in distance learning, more faculty than ever are "designing" Web-based courses. Faculty report that 37% serve as content designers, 20% manage information, and 41% of faculty design, deliver, and manage their own Web-based courses. Within this population, 53% of faculty spends more hours per week preparing and delivering distance learning courses than they do for comparable traditional courses (National Education Association, 2000). Fortunately, faculty is turning to the pedagogy of designing high-quality distance courses and academic programs. The need remains, however, to provide a theoretical foundation for design decisions made by faculty where fundamental assumptions, strategies, and practices align to the culture of the institution and the pragmatic and technological issues of using the Web as the vehicle for instructional delivery. Too often, designers of online curriculum are captivated by the technological capability of the Web without dealing with the underlying issues and key elements that may include context, tools to supplement and extend thinking, and pedagogical scaffolding (Hannafin & Land, 2000; Sherry, 1996).

A GRADUATE PROGRAM IN INSTRUCTIONAL TECHNOLOGY

The scenario that will be embedded throughout this paper is a description of a graduate program in instructional technology at a state institution that has not yet established a solid infrastructure for distance learning institution-wide. Students in the program represent a wide-range of professions to include classroom teachers, technology coordinators in schools and school systems, consultants from the multimedia and Web-based instruction industry, active military professionals engaged primarily in training and instructional design, health care workers engaged primarily in training and development of instructional materials, and a few social service employees. The common variable is that students want to apply innovative technologies to instructional and training situations with both adult and child learners.

The program's foundation is instructional systems design and psychological theories of learning. All other courses are built on this foundation. At present, innovative technologies including the design of multimedia instructional materials, Web-based instruction, electronic performance support systems, two-way interactive distance learning systems, and more are taught within the program.

The program is designed to accommodate the part-time student taking two courses a semester with courses clustered to promote authentic learning experiences. See Table 1 for a complete listing of courses and sequence.

The institution has not established an institution-wide organizational structure for distance learning, thus providing an opportunity to align the program in a way that best suits the learner, the learning outcomes, and the tools. In addition to establishing a program, pragmatic issues of administration such as student registration, online advising, financial aid, the library, and the bookstore had to be decided prior to program initiation. Additionally, the overarching infrastructure for supporting students in class had to be determined. Tutorials on how to be a distance learner had to be created simultaneously to the design of instructional materials. As well, mentors for each course were hired to assist the instructor in maintaining a solid feedback mechanism for students, especially as they embarked on the program for the first time. Much research went into the

TABLE 1. Program Courses and Sequence

Semester 1: Trends and Issues Conference for Instructional Technology	Semester 2: Constructing Learning	Semester 3: Policy and Development of Web-Based Instruction
Instructional Management and Technology (EDG 6344) Instructional Technology Seminar (EME 6812)	Principles of Instructional Design (EDG 5332) Application of Psychology Theories to Current Issues of Student Development and Learning (EDF 6211)	Web-based Instruction (EME 6414C) Analysis of Distance Education (EME 6458)
Semester 4: Multimedia Team 2000	Semester 5: Action Research in Instructional Technology	Semester 6: Planning for Technology Integration and Change
Multimedia Tools (EME 6415) Educational Theories and Practices: Social, Multicultural, Historical and Philosophical Analysis (EDF 6608)	Statistics (EDF 5404) Educational Research (EDF 6481)	Instructional Technology Planning and Change (EME 6607) Integrated Technology Learning Environments (EME 6408)

design of instructional materials that contained balanced amounts of both content and social interaction to ensure that learners were engaged in learning and motivated to continue in the program (Northrup, in press; Rasmussen & Northrup, 1999a; Northrup & Rasmussen, 2000). Fortunately, the technological infrastructure of the campus enabled the program designers to experiment with a range of presentation and communications tools along with streaming video and audio as needed.

Bridging the Gap Between Theory and Practice

It's difficult to prescribe one "best fit" for designing interactive online courses, given the wide range of communications and collaboration possibilities available on the World Wide Web. It is, however, important to *ground* the design of the learning environment in solid theory and pedagogy as distance learning has been criticized for having very little if any theoretical context (Moore, 1993). Hannafin, Hannafin, Land, and Oliver (1997) discuss *grounded design* as a context for dealing with the range of design decisions that best facilitate learning outcomes. Grounded design is defined as "the systematic implementation of processes and procedures that are rooted in established theory and research in human learning" (p. 102). Grounded design does not presume that one belief system is superior over another; it merely suggests alignment among the foundations, assumptions and methods selected (Northrup, in press).

GROUNDED DESIGN DECISIONS

Grounded design suggests alignment among foundations, assumptions and methods selected. It is presumed that courses comprising a Web-based program will have varying instructional strategies, as course outcomes will vary. However, establishing a framework for an entire program will provide much-needed consistency for both students and faculty. Within grounded design, five areas are emphasized to include: psychological, pedagogical, technical, cultural, and pragmatic. This paper will discuss each aspect of grounded design and will provide examples throughout of a graduate program in instructional technology that was built around this framework.

Psychological Grounding

The psychological aspect of grounded design emphasizes theory and research on how people learn. With theorists studying learning since the

1800s, there are many beliefs about the way people learn (Driscoll, 2000). Despite the differing philosophies of learning, theorists generally agree that learning is ". . . a persisting change in human performance potential . . . and that a change in performance or performance potential must come about as a result of a learner's experience and interaction with the world" (p. 11). Sherry (1996) suggests that two dominant views of learning have emerged, a more traditional, information processing approach and a constructivist approach. Driscoll promotes Cognitive Information Processing as an integration of a variety of perspectives where the human learner is conceived to be a processor of information, in much the same way that a computer processes information through input, storage, and output.

The alternative approach, constructivism, is based on the learner's active construction of knowledge as attempts are made to make meaning from experience. Constructivists emphasize learning in context, through meaningful activities that can be called upon again and again for relevant problem solving. Additionally, the content can be interpreted by the learner who is able to see more relationships and connections to complex, ill-structured tasks (Brown & Palincsar, 1989).

Based on the notion of situating learning in context, developers of the graduate program in instructional technology selected *situated cognition* as the primary construct primarily because knowledge and conditions of its use are linked in realistic contexts (Brown, Collins, & Duguid, 1989). Most courses were established within the framework of providing realistic contexts for learning. For example, a principles of instructional design course was offered in conjunction to a psychological foundations course with the context of designing instruction as the meaningful activity. The courses provide legitimate peripheral participation (Lave & Wegner, 1998) as their premise, with a performance support tool as the guide for the course along with practicing instructional designers posing real situations in which students are to work to resolve. Within each course cluster, a unique situation provides the context for the semester.

Pedagogical Grounding

The pedagogical aspect of grounded design presumes that the affordances and activities of the environment are aligned precisely to the psychological aspect of grounded design. Again, using the grounded design approach, the assumption is that one belief system is *not* superior over another; it merely suggests alignment among the foundations, assumptions and methods selected (Hannafin & Land, 2000).

In the graduate program in instructional technology, the psychological grounding in a more constructivist, student-centered environment suggests that authentic learning experiences that anchor instruction to real-world experiences be used. This allows for new knowledge to be connected to a learner's cognitive structure. In this learning environment, presented ideas are connected to a learner's existing knowledge system. Anchored instruction consists of meaningful learning experiences that students can extrapolate to their own professional demands as they integrate the new knowledge into their work environment (CTGV, 1991). Table 2 presents the design variables employed in the instructional technology graduate program that consider both psychological and pedagogical grounding.

Based on the theoretical and design framework, the instructional technology graduate program was constructed using a model of two courses per semester that are anchored in one context. Students are required to have access to the World Wide Web along with accompanying hardware/software required for the program. The following are design features of the program:

1. *Mentors* are assigned to individual students to provide content, heuristic, and technical support. The support inherent in these duties includes tasks such as: working with students to solve technology problems, interpreting lesson assignments as required, and being generally on call to solve other problems. Mentors are graduate students, either instructional technology majors or content experts who provide another avenue of access to online students. The key characteristic of a mentor is that of access–they must be available to students to minimize the frustrations naturally found in a Web-based environment. In addition, mentors must be active problem solvers, as every student will have slightly different problems than the others. Mentors do not fulfill the role of an instructor–they have no responsibilities for providing content nor do they grade student work. Mentors provide peer support to students to facilitate their success in a distance environment.

2. *Pairs of courses* delivered together are situated around one contextual learning experience. Students, for example, take the instructional systems design course at the same time they take the psychological foundations course. With this combination of

courses, students who are designing and developing instruction also apply the content knowledge developed during the psychological theories of instruction course. Table 1 outlines the program sequence.

3. *Cognitive Apprenticeship* exists through scaffolding and coaching of knowledge, heuristics, and strategy. Student-to-student, student-to-instructor, and student-to-instructional apprenticeship opportunities exist.

4. *Social Context* of the course is promoted by establishing learning communities that deal with rational problem solving, shared multiple perspectives, and reflection of works-in-progress. Much collaboration is designed into the program through the formation of study-buddy teams and the collaborative assignments posed to similar groups of learners. For example, a team of classroom teachers may investigate how to plan for technology integration in K-12, while another team is working collaboratively to determine how to integrate technology into the health-care industry. All groups socially negotiate their roles and responsibilities, while being held accountable, both as a group, and individually, for completion and sharing with other groups online.

Technical Grounding

This aspect of grounded design deals primarily with the influence of how media can support, constrain, or enhance a learning environment (Hannafin & Land, 2000). Given the possibilities of the Web, it is easy

TABLE 2. Design Variables in Program

Strategy	Rationale
Cognitive Apprenticeships	Faculty serve as knowledge experts
Modeling	Instructor actions serve as illustrations of good practice
Scaffolding	Learning supports are inherent in the instruction
Coaching/Mentoring	Tutoring and support in instructional practices and content
Collaboration	Group work and support
Authentic Context	Real-world scenarios
Authentic Activity	Real-world assignments
Reflection	Consideration and re-consideration of activities

to get lost in the newest fad online rather than contemplating how the technology can serve to structure the learning experience itself. Bearing in mind that the psychological, pedagogical, and technical aspects are interwoven, design decisions at this point are evident in the online learning experience itself. For example, if it is determined that learning should be socially constructed and that collaboration, communication, and interaction are all to be evidenced in the learning experience, a solid media selection decision can be made to make this occur. Technologies such as chat rooms, threaded discussion groups, and online whiteboards can be used to promote social construction of knowledge. Many times, designers take the inverse approach by selecting the media prior to considering the learning itself.

In the graduate instructional technology program, technical grounding was based on the assumptions of situated learning and anchored instruction. Given that learning is situated in real-world experience, it is essential for learners to have ongoing communications and collaboration online. Studies are beginning to show that students taking courses on the Web develop a stronger sense of community than those in traditional settings (Davidson-Shivers & Rasmussen, 1998, 1999), thus exacerbating need to promote collaboration, communications, and interaction online. To do this, a *communications structure* had to be in place along with providing technical support to eliminate wasted time. Primary to the assumptions are the anchoring of instructional components. Anchoring instruction is evidenced by providing case studies, goal-based scenarios, and activities in which learners engage in problem-solving through analysis, synthesis, and evaluation. In one example, Who Shot KR? the president of a multimedia design company has made promises to the client that are unrealistic. The promises impact the entire design team, from graphic artists to instructional designers and video producers. Each member of the team tries to reconcile the problems created by the company president thus creating a more realistic timeline for the completion of the multimedia product, while still staying within budget.

Technical decisions based on communications were made based on the *Communications Network* embedded within the program. The idea of communication and the related issues are the most critical element in the implementation of distance, Web-based programs. Many of the criticisms focused on distance education programs revolve around the perceived passive, isolated environment of the distant learner (Rasmussen & Northrup, 1999b). Open communication lines and active learning strategies assist in developing a learning community that is dynamic, everchanging, and positive. Interactive communication among different members of the community ensures that knowledge is constructed, that problems are averted, and that students continue to be motivated in the program.

There are a wide variety of communication networks found in the distance learning environment. The first communication network begins at the inception of the program where the instructor communicated with the designers and developers or technical support. During the class, instructors communicate with mentors who serve as liaisons with students and provide personalized, quick responses. Each mentor is responsible for 20-30 students, permitting instructors to work with larger numbers of students. Instructors also, naturally, interact with individual students, and the students as a class.

Mentors, in addition to communicating with instructors and students, must also work with other mentors and individuals who provide technical support. (Technical support staff supply answers to all kinds of technical problems.) In these activities, solutions to problems are developed and shared to minimize student and instructor frustrations. Mentors are guides and provide general support to give students advice and solutions. Mentors assist instructors in working with students, but do not interfere with the instructor's authority and responsibilities.

In a distance learning environment, students must be assisted in developing a learning community. Students need to "get to know" each other and be able to work with one another in large and small groups. To meet this challenge in distance environments, students must virtually meet classmates and develop strategies to work collectively at a distance. Peer-to-peer relationships must be encouraged as well as developing a class identity. Interactions among and between students facilitate this growth of community.

Cultural Grounding

This aspect of grounded design focuses on the prevailing values of the learning community itself. Hannafin and Land (2000) provide examples of medical schools promoting lab-intensive activity, while law schools promote a high level of case-based learning. Additionally, teacher education programs provide intensive practical experience while many instructional technology programs promote hands-on laboratory experience with intensive internships in the public and in the private sector. Institutionally and programmatically, online programs should reflect the culture of the campus-based program in this regard.

There is a certain level of comfort in maintaining the rigor of the institution from which the program is being provided.

With regard to the graduate instructional technology program, the campus-based program is applied in nature, as are all graduate programs in the college. Therefore, it is aligned to the psychological and pedagogical framework of learning in context. Given the nature of the college's population of returning students (many are mid-career professionals who are taking courses in the evenings and on weekends), the program must directly meet the needs of the adult learner. Part of the attraction of the program is its focus on application of newly learned knowledge in the job environment, with coaching and mentoring available as needed.

Pragmatic Grounding

This aspect of grounded design emphasizes reconciling available resources and constraints. When designing Web-based instruction, determining how to reconcile available resources is the trick, as most institutions of higher education do not have new funds to direct into distance learning. Many institutions choose to redirect money into distance learning, especially if there is a return-on-investment yielding more students in locations previously unable to attend graduate programs. As more institutions opt to deliver courses at a distance, competition for students will become an even more prominent factor for administrators to choose to implement distance learning.

Many pragmatic issues exist when designing Web-based programs, such as defining requirements for admissions, library, bookstore, financial obligations and registration. These administrative processes must be streamlined and coordinated to facilitate students' use of the system. Distance students are unable to physically walk from office to office to solve administrative problems. A one-stop support structure, along with staff who can make decisions, minimizes student frustrations and problems, as this system ensures that students continue in the program without ongoing administrative difficulties.

Additional pragmatic concerns include security, connectivity, troubleshooting and maintenance. Each must be addressed in order for the program to operate smoothly.

Security. The issues associated with security can be divided into two areas: access and administration. Comprehensive security access must provide instructors, students, and the design and development team with appropriate access to the course and program Web site. Confidential material (e.g., grades, tests, and students projects) as well as intellectual property must be protected, typically through the use of passwords. All authorized users of the site do not require equal access to information on the site. Development of an appropriate system requires the use of comprehensive site management programs such as WebCT or BlackBoard or the use of database-foundational software such as Cold Fusion or Oracle.

In addition to access, security issues also revolve around functions such as registration, fee payment, and other general issues of student support. Registration of students is critical for the continued success of programs and courses. Ensuring that student records remain accessible to authorized users, but confidential, is very important. Further, the fee payment for registered classes must be considered and issues of secure payment via the World Wide Web or other means must be addressed. Finally, aspects of student support, such as counseling, admissions, and financial aid must be kept in secure environments.

Solutions to security issues range from simple Java scripts on individual pages to complex programs on secure servers. These solutions are very dependent on the program, the needs of the instructors and students, and administrative requirements of the institution. Each educational situation will have different requirements that require various strategies of solutions.

Connectivity. Issues of how and when students connect to the distant program are also critical to ensuring student success and motivation as well as to facilitate communication among the learning community. Students must be able to access the site as well as receive student support as necessary. Server backups and regular monitoring of systems are needed for students, faculty, and mentors to be able to connect to technology tools.

Student support systems can be made up of a variety of elements, including: frequently asked questions (FAQ), program and course requirements, technical requirements, and strategies of successful distant learning techniques. Comprehensive support permits students to access the information that they need to remain connected to the learning environment.

Troubleshooting. Troubleshooting is divided into two areas: technical and instruction. Proactive troubleshooting techniques provide all users of the distance system with a reliable learning environment that is conducive to the process of teaching and learning. For the technical areas of troubleshooting, the Web site and needs of the instructor and student must be considered. The Web site requires an active, working site, so that it can be accessed, and graphics and links need to be active. Overall, the Web site needs to be functional and easy to use. Instructors and students also require support–the navigation should be clear, directions should be easy to follow, and the site should contain a central place for students to go for help.

The instruction needs to be reviewed and reexamined to ensure that it is aligned to the goals and objectives of the program and the course. In addition, test items need to be aligned to the objectives and the instruction. As the course continues, adjustments may need to be made to the course or to specific assignments. Being flexible as an instructor is key to the continued success of the learning environment.

Maintenance. Maintenance becomes equally important during the implementation of a course or program. Week-to-week implementation and modifications based on technological requirements and realities require continual monitoring of the learning environment. Maintenance issues, such as revising the instruction for new instructors and learners and revising links, become especially important as the program continues after initial implementation.

Instructors and mentors must monitor the learning environment closely to ensure that students receive answers to questions and continue to succeed in the program. Subsequent presentation of the course will require additional modifications and maintenance in order for the class to appear fresh and up-to-date (Rasmussen, Northrup, & Lee, 1997).

CONTINUOUS IMPROVEMENT

Ongoing, continuous improvement through formative evaluation ensures that the instruction meets the needs of the students and extends program quality. Several formative evaluation strategies exist that are useful in this context. Traditional one-to-one and small group evaluations proposed by Dick and Carey (1996) work extremely well if a small sample of the target audience is available for ongoing reviews. Dick and Carey propose that formative evaluation look specifically at student outcome and attitude data. With a one-to-one and small group evaluation, these data can be collected on an ongoing basis with constant modifications to the course content, aesthetics, and general issues related to the course. Additionally, using a rapid prototyping model to test ideas in stages will go a long way in reducing the overall time required to design and develop entire graduate programs.

CONCLUSION

Building innovative programs, based on a strong theoretical design, that support student performance and learning ensures that high-quality programs are able to deliver instruction to learners who are unable or unwilling to participate in traditional learning environments. The establishment of a framework to design and develop open-ended, yet grounded, environments enables programs to meet student needs and continue to provide superior learning environments.

REFERENCES

Brown, J. S., Collins, A., & Duguid, P. (1989). Situated cognition and the culture of learning. *Educational Researcher, 18*(1), 32-41.

Brown, J. S., & Palincsar, A. (1989). Guided, cooperative learning and individual knowledge acquisition. In L. B. Resnick (Ed.), *Knowing and learning: Essays in honor of Robert Glaser* (pp. 393-451). Hillsdale, NJ: Erlbaum.

Cognition and Technology Group at Vanderbilt (1991). Technology and the design of generative learning environments. *Educational Technology, 31*(5), 34-40.

Council for Higher Education Accreditation (2000). *Distance learning in higher education, CHEA Update, Number 2* [Online]. Available: *http://www.chea.org/Commentary/distance-learning-2.cfm*

Davidson-Shivers, G. V., & Rasmussen, K. (November, 1998). *Collaborative instruction on the Web: Students learning together.* Paper presented at the annual conference WebNet '98, Orlando, FL.

Davidson-Shivers, G. V., & Rasmussen, K. (February, 1999). *Mentoring: Apprenticeships for learning through the WWW.* Paper presented at the annual conference Association of Educational Communications and Technology, Houston, TX.

Dick, W., & Carey, L. (1996). *The systematic design of instruction* (4th ed.). New York: Harper-Collins.

Driscoll, M. P. (2000). *Psychology of learning for instruction* (2nd ed.). Needham Heights, MA: Allyn & Bacon.

Hannafin, M. J., Hannafin, K. M., Land, S. M., & Oliver, K. (1997). Grounded practice and the design of constructivist learning environments. *Educational Technology Research and Development, 44*(3).

Hannafin, M. J., & Land, S. M. (2000). Student-centered learning environments. In D. H. Jonassen and S. M. Land (Eds.), *Theoretical foundations of learning environments* (pp. 1-24). Mahwah, NJ: Erlbaum.

Lave, J., & Wegner, E. (1998). *Situated learning: Legitimate peripheral participation.* Cambridge, U.K.: University Press.

Moore, M. G. (1993). Theory of transactional distance. In D. Keegan (Ed.), *Theoretical principles of distance education.* New York: Routledge.

National Education Association (June 2000). *A survey of traditional and distance learning higher education members.* [Online]. Available: *http://www.nea.org/he*

Northrup, P. T. (in press). A framework for designing interactivity into Web-based instruction. *Educational Technology.*

Northrup, P. T., & Rasmussen, K. L. (2000). *Designing a Web-based program: Theory to design.* Paper presented at the annual conference of the Association for Educational Communications and Technology, Long Beach, CA.

Rasmussen, K. L., & Northrup, P. T. (February, 1999a). *Interactivity and the Web: Making and maintaining contact.* Paper presented at the annual conference Association of Educational Communications and Technology, Houston, TX.

Rasmussen, K. L., & Northrup, P.T. (1999b). *Strategies that facilitate instructor-student communication.* Paper presented at the annual conference Ed-Media '99 Seattle, WA.

Rasmussen, K. L., Northrup, P. T., & Lee, R. (1997). Implementing Web-based instruction. In B. H. Kahn (Ed.), *Web-based instruction* (pp. 341-346). Englewood Cliffs, NJ: Educational Technology Publications.

Sherry, L. (1996). Issues in distance learning. *International Journal of Educational Telecommunications, 1*(4), 337-365.

Guglielmo Trentin

Designing Online Education Courses

SUMMARY. The aim of this article is to focus on the main elements that characterize online course design, a process usually comprising two strictly related macro-phases: the course plan itself and the communication architecture for the development and running of the proposed learning activities.

The article addresses the impossibility of designing an online course on the basis of criteria typical of onsite education, and emphasizes the importance of adopting methods and strategies that are compatible with the technological medium and the communication dynamics to which it gives rise.

The suggestions that will be made are not intended to represent a codified formula for the design of online courses, but rather to provide discussion points on key issues within the process. *[Article copies available for a fee from The Haworth Document Delivery Service: 1-800-342-9678. E-mail address: <getinfo@haworthpressinc.com> Website: <http://www.HaworthPress.com> © 2001 by The Haworth Press, Inc. All rights reserved.]*

KEYWORDS. Distance education, course design, computer mediated communication, computer conferencing

GUGLIELMO TRENTIN is Professor, Instituto Tecnologie Didattiche, Consiglio Nazionale delle Ricerche, Via De Marini 6, 16149 Genova, Italia (E-mail: trentin@itd.ge.cnr.it).

[Haworth co-indexing entry note]: "Designing Online Education Courses." Trentin, Guglielmo. Co-published simultaneously in *Computers in the Schools* (The Haworth Press, Inc.) Vol. 17, No. 3/4, 2001, pp. 47-66; and: *The Web in Higher Education: Assessing the Impact and Fulfilling the Potential* (ed: Cleborne D. Maddux, and D. LaMont Johnson) The Haworth Press, Inc., 2001, pp. 47-66. Single or multiple copies of this article are available for a fee from The Haworth Document Delivery Service [1-800-342-9678, 9:00 a.m. - 5:00 p.m. (EST). E-mail address: getinfo@haworthpressinc.com].

47

A wide spectrum of possibilities exists for the educational use of ICT (Information and Communication Technologies). These run from using the Web as an online tool for seeking out and distributing learning material up to the organization and management of virtual classes using the online education approach. These can be grouped under three separate headings:

1. *Educational processes based on onsite teaching*, where the Internet is used to gain remote access to learning material, with the possible addition of online counseling from tutors.
2. *Mixed educational processes (online/onsite)*, which combine characteristics of onsite education (lectures, group work, etc.) and of online education (discussion, remotely guided exercises, etc.), and where activities of either kind complement those of the other.
3. *Wholly online educational processes*, that include no onsite activities at all, being based on distance interaction between the actors in the process (students, tutors, experts, etc.) carried out using both asynchronous communication (e-mail, computer conferencing, etc.) and synchronous communication (chatting, audio/video conferencing, etc.).

This paper will concentrate on the design of courses that fall into this last category and that adopt approaches identified with so-called *third-generation distance education*, otherwise known as *online education* (Harasim, 1990; Nipper, 1989).

THIRD-GENERATION DISTANCE EDUCATION

In the field of distance learning, systems defined as third-generation are those based on intense interaction between all the players in the process with the purpose of forming a collaborative learning community, albeit a virtual one.

In traditional distance courses (those known as *first-* and *second-generation* courses, or, alternatively, *correspondence* and *multimedia* courses) the emphasis is less on the communication element than on individual exploitation of learning material. By contrast, in online education, it is the collaboration among participants that stimulates and fosters learning.

Communicating at a distance, participants discuss the course content and/or engage in practical activities like producing reports, designing projects, and so on. The attendees swap ideas on the course subject; and in this way, the whole group can share and benefit from the experience of each participant, thus gaining fresh insight into the particular course content (Kaye, 1991). This is done with the assistance of tutors, who support participant-participant and participant-content interaction (Berge, 1995). Courses based on this model are run by staff with expertise in three different areas: contents, online course methodology, and technological aspects. In some cases, different staff members handle these areas separately; while in others, they are covered by the same person.

The tutors' work is complemented by one or more content experts, who are mainly involved in the phase of course design but may also be accessible online while the course is in progress (though this is not normally the case). Accordingly, there is a need for the roles of all the players in the learning process to be clearly defined (Trentin & Scimeca, 1999). The experts usually look after course content and its structuring, outline activities, and sometimes suggest the most suitable educational strategies for achieving learning goals.

Once the content structure has been defined and the type of learning activities decided, the tutor has the task of reshaping the course plan devised by the experts, drawing upon online education strategies in order to make the course work on the net.

DESIGNING AN ONLINE COURSE

When dealing with online education, it is necessary to rethink the methodologies, criteria, and approaches normally adopted for conventional educational design/planning. Account must be made for the positive and negative influence of ICT use, which can be attributed to a number of specific factors such as the particular type of communication (chiefly text-based, but also video communication); the shift in the teacher's role within the class; and, last but not least, problems involved in managing student access to network resources.

The design of an online course may be divided into two strictly correlated and interconnected macro-phases: the *course plan* itself and the *communication architecture* for the development and management of the learning activities that the course envisages.

ONLINE EDUCATION: THE COURSE PLAN

There are a host of different approaches for designing online courses: We shall propose just one–that adopted in the design of the Polaris courses (Trentin, 1997a) for in-service teacher training.

The various steps in the design process (see Appendix A) will be listed in order, although each may actually have a retroactive effect on the one that precedes it.

Design Constraints

At the outset, it is advisable to define the constraints and limits within which the course is to operate. These may concern:

1. Economic aspects
2. The contexts of reference (higher education, pre/in-service training, etc.)
3. The profile of the participants and the conditions surrounding their participation
4. The type of technology to be used
5. The type of support that the course provider can offer students
6. The period in which the course will be held
7. The availability of experts for online consultation
8. The feasibility of producing ad hoc learning material

In a way, the constraints delimit the area in which the subsequent design phases will develop.

Analysis and Definition of Learning Needs

A distance course can either be pre-packaged and offered to a given population or produced on commission (tailor-made courses). In any case, its aims and objectives cannot be defined without first carrying out a detailed study of the users' learning needs and then setting them out in detail.

The design of pre-packaged courses begins with a study of the learning needs of a specific user group, and this provides the basis for putting together the package. In the case of tailor-made courses, the users themselves express their learning needs to the course designers.

Definition of Aims

The aims are usually defined in terms of the hopes expressed by those who propose or commission the course: *"the students will learn how to . . . they will realize that . . . they will get used to . . . they will be able to . . . they will distinguish between . . . ,"* etc. So the objectives need to be formulated in terms of *"gaining awareness of . . . learning to use tools to . . . analyzing and comparing . . . ,"* etc. Essentially, the transition from defining aims to setting objectives centers on identifying learning activities that allow measurement of the degree to which aims/objectives have been reached (Rowntree, 1981).

Defining and Structuring Objectives

Proper definition of objectives has a strong impact on the subsequent design phases and especially on the mechanism used to evaluate both the course as a whole and learning in particular. In most cases, it is worth operating at two different levels, namely, the definition of final and intermediate objectives. The former case normally sees the simultaneous involvement of tutors (those who coordinate the project and act as moderators among the course commissioners, experts, students, etc.) and experts (those who provide the content expertise). By contrast, in the definition of intermediate objectives the leading role is played by content experts, with the aid of tutors, who have ultimate responsibility for guiding the students toward the pre-set goals.

Structuring of objectives may be carried out in a variety of manners, including arrangement in a taxonomy (Bloom, 1956) or in a hierarchy of main and subordinate objectives (Gagné, 1970). Figure 1 shows an example of a hierarchy.

It is often advisable to try to draft the intermediate and final evaluation tests for the course immediately following initial definition of objectives; in other words, before proceeding with the subsequent phases of course design. This is a very effective way of gaining feedback about the consistency of the structure of the objectives (Trentin, 1997b).

Course Prerequisites

At this point, before passing on to defining and structuring course content, it is necessary to identify the knowledge and basic skills that students will need in order to participate in course activities.

FIGURE 1. Structure of Objectives in a Course on the Use of ICT in Education

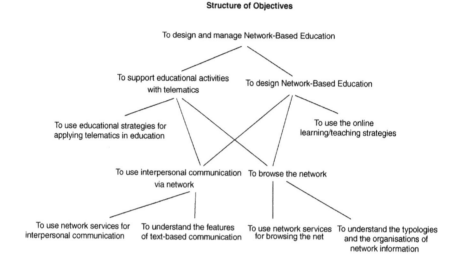

At the university level these relate to current year, course of study, and the student's effective knowledge both of the content and the technology to be used, elements which can easily be gauged through an entrance exam.

When it comes to distance education, however, the problem is far more complex, given the certain non-homogeneity of the student group. The need therefore arises for fully-fledged pre-testing in order to define an average profile of the virtual class that is to be constructed. When forming student groups, it is always important to seek the most homogeneous level possible of pre-knowledge and skills, all the more so when dealing with an online course.

Defining the prerequisites is therefore a crucial step for course designers, as it helps them to establish a kind of substratum of subordinate knowledge, the foundations for the scaffolding that will support knowledge acquisition during the course. What's more, defining the prerequisites is also important for setting the course entry conditions.

But how can these prerequisites be defined? The course designers (experts and tutors) can define them in terms of the course objectives, or they can be gleaned from a preliminary study of the population of potential course beneficiaries.

Content Structuring

The sound structuring of online course content into main and subordinate topics is strongly advised, given the close connection this structure has with the structure of the Web-based environment that is to host the learning activities and manage communication flow. If sound prior structuring of objectives is done upstream (using the hierarchy approach, for example), then the corresponding content structure will result almost automatically.

Online courses are usually divided into stages, each of which is further divided into a series of modules. The course topic is consequently subdivided into general sections, some of which are necessary introductions to other sections, while others are optional or designed for supplementary study.

In this phase, too, the teaming up of content experts and tutors plays a key role. Thanks to their knowledge of the subject area, the content experts are able to define a structure suitable for the pursuit of the learning objectives. On the other hand, the tutors bring their know-how in designing and running online courses and are aware of how a given content structure can be adapted to network use. There is a possibility (indeed a high likelihood) that the experts involved will be unacquainted with the concept of online education; and, consequently, they are likely to produce a content structure based on a traditional teaching approach.

Referring back to Figure 1, at this point each node of the hierarchy ought to be associated to content that will lead toward the achievement of the related learning objective. The outcome is shown in Figure 2.

Course Flexibility

Online courses, especially those based on collaborative strategies, must take proper account of participants' specific needs. Course flexibility is called for in response to a variety of factors: differences in equipment levels, differences in the amount of free time available to dedicate to the course, differences in the level of know-how in the technology to be used, and so on.

A solution that has proved effective here is to draw on the dual-track concept and provide a mainstream channel together with alternative pathways for supplementary study. To put it briefly, an online course should comprise:

1. A main path to be followed by all participants that leads towards the achievement of a pre-established minimum number of learning objectives.

2. A series of optional paths, some of which are outlined in the design phase, while others are devised to meet needs that arise as the course unfolds–always bearing in mind the ultimate aims of the course. Clearly, these optional paths are recommended for those participants (or groups thereof) who get through the main path activities before the others, either because they had more time to dedicate to the tasks or had a stronger grasp of the subject from the outset. These supplementary paths are also useful for participants who wish to form virtual subgroups in order to investigate topics that fall ouside the original course plan.

FIGURE 2. The Content Structure in a Course on the Use of ICT in Education

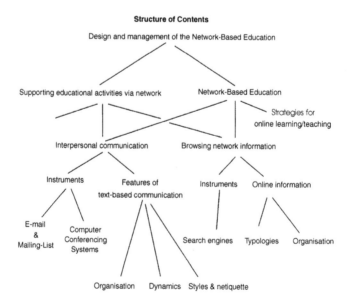

In this respect it is vital to define clearly these optional activities and to decide under what conditions they are to be proposed. In any case, they are not to be considered as substitutes for sections of the main path.

Choice of Educational Strategies

Having defined the educational objectives, we need to identify the learning strategies to be adopted for their pursuit. These may include instructional training (in the use of tools and services), exercises, discussion, collaborative work, simulation, role-playing or tutorials, to name but a few.

It is important to identify the most effective methodology for employing each of these strategies. For instance, there are a number of options available for employing collaborative learning, including strategies like reciprocal teaching (Palincsar & Brown, 1984) and the jigsaw method (Aroson, 1978).

In any case, the identification of educational strategies calls for a modicum of awareness of what network interaction involves, of the dynamics of computer mediated communication, and thus of the various degrees of effectiveness that those strategies may have at different moments in online activity. This means that the classroom experience that a teacher/trainer has gained over the years provides no guarantee of success when working in online education, especially the first time out.

Defining Evaluation Criteria

The complicated matter of defining evaluation criteria is still the subject of research. Evaluating an online course raises a number of problems at different levels. Two in particular are of special significance:

1. Evaluation of learning
2. Evaluation of student participation levels in terms of activity carried out online

Evaluation of learning. Without going into detail about the modes normally used for evaluating learning in an online course, it should nevertheless be stressed that their definition must go hand in hand with the definition of educational objectives and of the educational strategies employed for pursuing those objectives. What this means is that the learning strategy itself often suggests the mode of evaluation. For instance, a strategy that features online discussion calls for evaluation based on qualitative-quantitative analysis of the messages produced by the participants (Henri, 1992; Thorpe, 1998).

Evaluation of participation levels. We need to distinguish here between two different ways of organizing participants: namely, virtual classes or learning circles (Riel, 1992). Virtual classes bring together individual participants who are scattered over a geographical area and therefore remote from one another. Learning circles, on the other hand, are locally based groups (e.g., students at the same university) who use ICT to communicate with other such groups situated in other geographical areas.

Evaluation of participation levels within virtual classes may be performed by analyzing the messages produced and by examining the log files to gauge the level of online "presence." (Log files are files in which the computer conferencing system automatically records each individual action that participants perform online: reading/writing messages, chatting activity, connection times, etc.). Evaluating the performance of members belonging to a learning circle is a far more difficult task, as online output generally reflects the activity of the group as a whole. A possible solution in such cases is (on at least one occasion during the course) to split up local groups and create new virtual groups made up of members from the various original groups, who will thus be forced to communicate exclusively online. This represents an effective way of singling out the members of local groups.

Furthermore, with both virtual and local groups it is important to define monitoring modes that will reveal to the tutors whether and to what extent the participants are focusing on the key issues as identified by the content experts. What's more, during the course the tutors should also be in a position to judge whether collaborative activity is actually taking place. As to the focus on key issues, a possible answer may be to agree with the content expert on a sort of checklist of key issues that participants must cover in their messages, and also to decide what level of detail ought to be reached. Ascertaining collaborative activity, on the other hand, can be done by using a simple double-entry grid (sender/receiver) to see whether there is cross-referenced communication among participants (quotes, questions and answers, etc.).

Defining Course Activities and Related Resources

Having chosen the educational strategies and methodologies, we can now go on and define course activities for putting these into action. We need to distinguish here between activities based on individual action and those that envisage collaborative learning, as well as between activities designed for use by virtual classes or by learning circles.

In addition, we need to indicate the resources required for each activity. These include learning and support material, course guides, available experts, the roles of the tutor (counselor, discussion moderator, facilitator for exercise activities or collaborative production, etc.), management modes for group activities, the network services to be used, etc.

On the question of material, it is useful to distinguish between what is already available (material used in previous courses or contained in books, articles, Web pages, courseware, etc.) and what needs to be produced especially for the course. In the latter case, attention needs to be paid to how one produces learning material for online courses, especially Web-based ones, but we will bypass this matter as it falls outside the scope of this paper.

Mode of Operation

When organizing network activities, it is crucial to decide how many participants are to be involved and how their interaction is to be organized (Webb, 1982; Riel & Levin, 1990). Accordingly, careful attention must be paid to setting the size of the virtual class in response to the activities proposed during the course and the role to be played by experts and each member of the tutoring staff while the course is underway.

Setting the Size of Online Study Groups

The considerations made below refer in a general manner to a situation in which there is a single entity at the other end of the telephone line, without distinguishing for the moment whether that entity is an individual course participant or a group of participants organized in a learning circle. In fact, from the viewpoint of network interaction, the local group is seen at a general level as a single entity that communicates with other entities (other local groups), all of whom are organized in learning circles.

This is an important consideration when defining the tutor-to-participant ratio which, ideally, should range from about one-to-ten to one-to-fifteen. This ratio, however, is a purely indicative one, given that the tutor's capacity to interact with a certain number of participants depends on the type of activity that he/she is called upon to run (discussion, exercises, role play, collaborative production, etc.). For the same reason, the size of the groups into which the participant population is divided is determined by the need to make their distance work efficient. For instance, if the students are to engage in collaborative production, they ought to be divided into small groups: Mediating online, especially via asynchronous communication, is never an easy task, as the longer discussion and decision-making go on, the more complex and time-consuming the collaboration will be.

Now let's look at the relationship between the type of activity and the size of the learning group. For simplicity's sake, we shall examine the cases of collaborative production and topic-based discussion.

Production Groups

The first point to make here is that collaborative production calls for a limited number of participants while discussion does not (remembering that it is best not to involve too many participants in any online activity). The reason is clear. Production activities involve continuous mediation between those working on the creation of a product: The more ideas are put forward, the harder the joint decision-making process becomes. What's more, when participants communicate in an asynchronous mode, the whole process slows down and this often undermines collaboration.

A reasonable number of participants might be somewhere around five to six units, remembering that a unit may represent a single individual interacting remotely with others or a local learning circle.

The size of virtual groups also depends on the type of collaborative strategy we intend to set in motion, as well as on the participants' specific situation regarding logistics and equipment. We need to decide whether to adopt a parallel strategy, whereby each group member works independently on a specific part of the overall product, or a reciprocal strategy, whereby each person contributes to each part of the overall product (Diaper & Sanger, 1993).

So the size of the groups into which participants are divided is governed by the need to maximize the efficiency of the distance work.

Discussion Groups

In the case of discussion groups, the situation is somewhat different: The more participants there are, the easier it is for ideas, observations, opinions, and so on, to circulate. When organizing online discussions, we often refer to the so-called "critical mass" (i.e., the minimum number of participants needed for a lively exchange).

But care needs to be taken here as well, because if the number of what we might call "active" participants exceeds a certain threshold, there is a risk of creating online "noise" that could damage the whole system. We might set the minimum number of dialoguing entities needed to guarantee a lively online discussion at about 10 to 12 units.

That said, those who frequent topical mailing lists and newsgroups may well object that this number is far too low. However, it has to be recognized that we are not talking about open discussions that anyone can join, take part in, and leave as they wish (as is the case with the aforementioned Internet services). Rather, we are dealing with groups that are aware they belong to a learning community that has set rules, planned and scheduled activities, and clearly defined procedures.

Defining Staff Members' Roles

Harmonization of staff members' roles is a key factor in the success of an online course. It helps to avoid overlap in the tutors' actions (which is often disorienting for the participants), to prevent clashes in the replies given by different tutors, to delineate the respective fields of action of the tutors and experts, to establish decision-making procedures, and so on.

One way of organizing the tutoring staff is as follows:

1. Assign each participant a *personal tutor* who will follow the student from close range throughout the whole course, giving advice, offering support when difficulties arise, etc.
2. Appoint a *head tutor* (sometimes called an *area tutor*) for each module of the course, someone who is to coordinate all the activities within his/her module, keep activities on schedule, support interaction between participants and the area expert (using different strategies according to whether that expert is available online or not), etc. In other words, this person acts as a reference tutor for that particular segment of the course.
3. Appoint a *head of staff*, a kind of course director, who is to supervise course activities, set the schedule, act as staff spokesperson when participants require explanation of course contents or methods, take the final decision on any eventuality arising during the course, etc.

Structure and Schedule of the Online Course

Online courses require careful prior structuring, given that once they are underway it becomes extremely hard to make substantial alterations. The same meticulous planning must also go into the scheduling of each individual activity, be it at the stage or the module level.

Outlining the schedule for the whole course is no easy task. No matter how much care and effort are put into estimating the time necessary for the various activities, the need invariably arises for constant calibration, ever-greater flexibility, and response to needs that come up throughout the course. All of this is inevitable given the asynchronous nature of communication between the participants and the freedom of the individual (or local group) to decide when to dedicate time to the course.

Nevertheless, there is a clear need, at least at the activity planning level, for general scheduling guidelines (i.e., markers for measuring the progress of the various activities and for deciding whether to readjust the timetable–which is usually the case).

Organizing the course into main and sub-activities is often useful on this count.

ONLINE EDUCATION:
THE COMMUNICATION ARCHITECTURE

Once the course design has been completed and the activities for the various players (students, tutors, experts, specialists, etc.) have been defined, the next step is the so-called logical structuring of the communication between the participants (i.e., outlining the system that is to guarantee proper flow of information and interpersonal exchange within the learning community). There are three main steps involved.

1. Identifying Communication Requirements

Online courses generally feature three main types of communication flow: between tutors (coordination and decision making); between tutors and experts (consultation and support); and within the various learning activities envisaged (among tutors, students, and experts).

Each of these flow types includes not only interpersonal communication, but also the exchange of documents and more generally of any material in electronic format.

In the first two cases, the communication requirements are fairly clear-cut and in a way quite easy to define. The last case is more complicated, in that the communication needs strictly depend on factors like the type of activity envisioned for the students, the educational strategy and methodology for their development, the breakdown of students into groups and subgroups, and so on. Consequently, for each activity proposed, the mode of interaction between all the players needs to be carefully examined.

2. Choosing the Most Suitable Network Services

Once the communication requirements have been defined, the next step is to choose the most suitable network service for running the course. This means assessing not just the performance of the chosen service but also the cost it entails: Cost differences exist between services of the same type (e.g., interpersonal communication, information access and sharing, etc.).

If the need is to organize, say, a discussion, the choice lies between a mailing list, which is virtually cost free, or a conference area within a computer conferencing system, where the technological and man-hour costs are undoubtedly greater. Similarly, document and material sharing can be handled either in a very rudimentary manner using file attachments on e-mail messages, or in a neater, more refined way by setting up a Web site.

3. Designing a Logical Communication Structure

Once the most suitable and affordable network services have been identified, the next step is designing the logical communication structure (i.e., organizing the interaction flows between the participants and arranging the shared information space) (Trentin, 1997c).

A number of issues will need to be tackled here. For example, how should the computer conferencing environments be divided into areas and subareas in accordance with the various learning activities (discussions, collaborative work, exercises, etc.)? If we opt to use mailing lists only, what lists should be organized and for which interpersonal communication activities? How can we go about arranging the course materials and the workgroups' in-progress products and displaying them on "electronic bookshelves"?

Furthermore, it is advisable, where possible, to provide areas outside those strictly dedicated to course activities. These may include so-called "cafés," where the participants can chat freely among themselves; an area for exchanging materials not strictly related to the course; a bulletin board for notices of different kinds, and a technical support area.

Clearly, using environments that can easily be tailored to communication requirements will make participation by the various players in the learning process all the more pleasant and straightforward.

It is worth examining the effects that may sometimes be obtained by prior subdivision of a communication environment into conferences and sub-conferences, and by the remodeling of that structure on the part of the course managers (tutors, teachers, etc.) while the course is underway (Trentin, 1998).

To get a clearer idea of this matter, let's imagine a book, or rather its contents page. By dividing the text into chapters and paragraphs and arranging them in a particular order, the author communicates to the reader his/her individual view of the topic structure at hand, and suggests a way of exploring it. In the same way, dividing an online learning environment into areas and subareas helps to channel the communication within the structure itself. In other words, it gives a glimpse of the vision that the course author has of the topic being dealt with.

It is therefore plain to see just how important it is for the online course manager to be skilled in designing the logical communication structure, especially in view of the dynamics that this structure will tend to instill as the course progresses (unforeseen supplementary study, organization of subgroups, etc.).

Let's take an example. Let's suppose that the participants in an online course (or some of them, at least) manifest particular interest in a subtopic of the main discussion theme and that, accordingly, the course manager opens a specific forum (a sub-conference in the computer conferencing system) for developing that subtopic. The participants often interpret such a move as a go-ahead, if not outright encouragement, to explore that subtopic, which may not have been foreseen during course designing.

DESIGN EVALUATION

The life cycle of a learning process can be broken down into three macro-phases–*design, execution*, and *validation*–where the later phases are often affected by the preceding ones. For instance, execution and validation often provide useful hints for improving or even redesigning the course.

The aim of this paper has been to analyze the design phase; and, therefore in conclusion, it is worth considering on what basis we might evaluate the success of that process. The most immediate answer would appear to be the extent to which the course goals have been reached (e.g., learning of given contents).

However, the achievement of educational objectives does not in itself mean that the course design is valid, although it is a necessary condition for declaring that a course has been successfully designed. This is because any design faults that become apparent while the course is underway may be patched up by the tutors. Thus, the direct monitoring of course activities becomes one of the main tools for evaluating the soundness of design decisions, not to mention the efficacy of the tutors' and experts' performance. Accordingly, monitoring should be orchestrated in such a way as to give feedback on all of the elements considered during the design phase.

Table 1 shows a possible checklist compiled on the basis of the preceding discussion.

TABLE 1. Checklist for Designing an Online Course and Communication Architecture

---

Online Course Design
Has sufficient consideration been given to project constraints?
Have the prerequisites for course participation been defined properly?
Have the stated objectives been reached? If not, why not?
Has the structure of the contents helped in reaching objectives?
Has flexibility helped to tailor the course to the participants' real learning needs?
Have the learning strategies and methodologies helped in reaching educational goals?
Have the activities proposed to the participants helped in applying the learning strategies?
Were the virtual groups of a suitable size for the proposed activities?
Did the learning materials and technologies prove effective and easy to use?
Were the course activities scheduled properly?
Did the tutoring staff offer satisfactory support?
Did the experts perform effectively?
Were there any interaction problems between the tutoring staff and the experts?
Did the modes for evaluating the participants prove effective for measuring learning and participation levels?
Design of the Communication Architecture
Were the communication flows for carrying out course activities correctly foreseen?
Were the most suitable network services chosen?
Did the logical communication structure respond properly to the participants' needs for interaction and exchange of material?

CONCLUSIONS

This article has repeatedly stressed the point that it is impossible to design an online course on the basis of criteria typical of onsite education and that it is necessary to adopt a series of methods and strategies that take into account the medium and the communication dynamics it triggers. Accordingly, the fundamental points in online education are:

1. Employing the most suitable ICT tools and methods to meet the requirements for interaction and exchange between all the players in the learning process.
2. Being aware of the (positive and negative) influence that the use of ICT can have on a range of factors like the particular type of communication (text-based or audio/videocommunication), the change in the teacher's role within the class and, last but not least, the problems involved in managing student access to network resources.

This awareness forms the basis for planning the design phases of an online course. Some of these have been examined in this paper, grouped under two general headings: *online course design* and the *communication architecture* for carrying out the course. Appendix A sets out and summarizes the relationships between the various elements that make up an online education project.

The structuring of the communication environment can influence the development of an online course and, therefore, it is important for the course designer to be fully versed not only in the technology to be used but also in the learning methodology.

Finally, on the basis of the so-called categorization of project elements, a possible checklist has been provided to help in the evaluation of the design process of an online course.

REFERENCES

Aroson, E. (1978). *The jigsaw classroom*. Beverly Hills, CA: Sage.

Berge, Z.L. (1995). Facilitating computer conferencing: Recommendations from the field. *Educational Technology, 35*(1), 22-29.

Bloom, B.S. (Ed.). (1956). *Taxonomy of educational objectives: Cognitive domain*. New York: McKay.

Diaper, D., & Sanger, C. (Eds.). (1993). *CSCW in practice: An introduction and case study*. London: Springer-Verlag.

Gagné, R. (1970). *The conditions of learning*. New York: Holt, Reinhart & Winston.

Harasim, L.M. (1990). *Online education: Perspectives on a new environment*. New York: Praeger.

Henri, F. (1992). Computer conferencing and content analysis. In A.R. Kaye (Ed.), *Collaborative learning through computer conferencing* (pp. 117-136). Berlin: Springer-Verlag.

Kaye, A.R. (1991). Learning together apart. In A. Kaye (Ed.), *Proceedings of the NATO advanced research workshop on collaborative learning and computer conferencing: Vol. 90. Computer and system sciences*. Berlin: Springer-Verlag.

Nipper, S. (1989). Third generation distance learning and computer conferencing. In R.D. Mason & A.R. Kaye (Eds.), *Mindweave: Communication, computers and distance education* (pp. 63-73). Oxford: Pergamon Press.

Palincsar, A., & Brown, A.L. (1984). Reciprocal teaching of comprehension-fostering and comprehension-monitoring. *Educational Psychologist, 20*, 167-183.

Riel, M., & Levin, J. (1990). Building electronic communities: Success and failure in computer working. *Instructional Science, 19*, 145-169.

Riel, M. (1992). A functional analysis of educational telecomputing: A case study of learning circles. *Interactive Learning Environments, 2*(1), 15-29.

Rowntree, D. (1981). *Developing courses for students*. Maidenhead, Berkshire: McGraw-Hill.

Thorpe, M. (1998). Assessment and "third generation" distance education. *Distance Education, 19*(2), 265-286.

Trentin, G. (1997a). Telematics and online teacher training: The Polaris project. *International Journal of Computer Assisted Learning, 13*(4), 261-270.

Trentin, G. (1997b). Computerized adaptive tests and formative assessment. *International Journal of Educational Multimedia and Hypermedia, 6*(2), 201-220.

Trentin, G. (1997c). Logical communication structures for network-based education and tele-teaching. *Educational Technology, 37*(4), 19-25.

Trentin, G. (1998). Computer conferencing systems seen by a designer of online courses. *Educational Technology, 38*(3), 36-43.

Trentin, G., & Scimeca, S. (1999). The roles of tutors and experts in designing online education courses. *Distance Education, 20*(1), 144-161.

Webb, N.M. (1982). Student interaction and learning in small groups. *Review of Educational Research, 52*(3), 421-445.

APPENDIX A

Online Education: Project Elements

Steven J. Coombs
Jillian Rodd

Using the Internet
to Deliver Higher Education:
A Cautionary Tale
About Achieving Good Practice

SUMMARY. This article reviews the development and delivery of a Higher Education course module as part of a large European University's Integrated Masters Program operating through a regional network of Rural Area Training and Information Opportunities (RATIO) telematic centres. The aim of the project was to provide remote learners living in the southwest of England with computer-supported solutions to access higher education as part of a technology-assisted distance education program. The module represented a shift from traditional educational delivery systems by using instructional courseware via an Internet Web site. Personal communications with module participants were conducted with the use of e-mail and videoconferencing information technology (IT) resources. Out of the original sixteen participants who enrolled in this Masters course module, four actually completed the learning sessions and two submitted final assignments. This article considers the key lessons

STEVEN J. COOMBS is Assistant Professor, School of Education, Sonoma State University, 1801 East Cotati Avenue, Rohnert Park, CA 94928-3609 (E-mail: steven. coombs@sonoma.edu).
JILLIAN RODD is Faculty of Arts and Education, University of Plymouth, Douglas Avenue, Exmouth, EX8 2AT, Devon, United Kingdom (E-mail: j1rodd@plymouth. ac.uk).

[Haworth co-indexing entry note]: "Using the Internet to Deliver Higher Education: A Cautionary Tale About Achieving Good Practice." Coombs. Steven J., and Jillian Rodd. Co-published simultaneously in *Computers in the Schools* (The Haworth Press, Inc.) Vol. 17. No. 3/4, 2001, pp. 67-90; and: *The Web in Higher Education: Assessing the Impact and Fulfilling the Potential* (ed: Cleborne D. Maddux, and D. LaMont Johnson) The Haworth Press. Inc., 2001, pp. 67-90. Single or multiple copies of this article are available for a fee from The Haworth Document Delivery Service [1-800-342-9678, 9:00 a.m. - 5:00 p.m. (EST). E-mail address: getinfo@haworthpressinc.com].

learned from this attrition rate and shares the mainly positive experiences of the remote tutor and the students engaged in this initiative. The implications regarding the use of the Internet for delivering higher education course modules through online distance learning are discussed in the light of cautions learned from this research project and important practical recommendations for future practice are made. *[Article copies available for a fee from The Haworth Document Delivery Service: 1-800-342-9678. E-mail address: <getinfo@haworthpressinc.com> Website: <http://www. HaworthPress.com> © 2001 by The Haworth Press, Inc. All rights reserved.]*

KEYWORDS. Telelearning, telematics, webministration, cyber-protocols, cybervoid, action research, synchronous and asynchronous communications systems, technical and pedagogic protocols

The key purpose of this research project was to take advantage of the opportunities offered by the Rural Area Training and Information Opportunities (RATIO) initiative and create an experimental Web site through which to offer a United Kingdom (UK) masters degree module. Because it was considered that students who were interested in IT might be attracted to such a format, it was decided to develop a module that already contained a high IT content. Thus, "IT for Personal Development and Project Management" was chosen as an appropriate module for conversion into telematic courseware. Telematics is a European word constructed from the terms "Telecommunications" and "Informatics" to express this new form of IT-assisted telelearning. This IT module was therefore considered to be suited for development as a distance learning program via a telematic platform that provides dissemination and assessment services through interactive student participation. Participants would have access to appropriate IT facilities located at the selected adult education RATIO centres across the southwestern region of the UK that have been set up from European Union (EU) funds. Careful developments of both *technical* and *pedagogic protocols* that underpin the delivery of telematic-assisted higher education programs were identified and summarized in Table 1. These protocols were needed to establish the effective use of such technology for remote learners following the academic task criteria for all masters' modules.

These tasks require learners to acquire academic skills covering the following five assessment areas:

1. Critical review of a body of knowledge.
2. Data collection and analysis.

3. Developing practice through a project.
4. Reflecting on practice.
5. Making an argument.

All of these areas are underpinned by deep criteria where the learner is expected to demonstrate abilities covering personal skills that involve research and investigation; organization and preparation; appropriateness of medium and process; practical competence; coherence; legibility; inventiveness and independence of thought; understanding of relevant historical, critical and cultural contexts; and, critical evaluation.

The challenge of this pilot project was to ensure that the technology-assisted module developed was capable of fulfilling the learning requirements outlined above through action research field-testing of the telematic resources developed with a small group of remote learners. The experiences of these remote learners were collected in order to evaluate the effectiveness of the technology adopted and the online distance education delivery systems implemented. Qualitative analysis of these action research findings was used to determine whether the professional development learning needs of the participants, relative to achievement of the five tasks, were achieved, and, if not, what lessons could be learned regarding future improvements. As this project represented a first attempt to integrate learning technologies into the main thrust of the integrated masters program, its development has been initially restricted to the creation of Web site courseware for one module. Academic communications support has been provided in the form of *synchronous* videoconference seminars and tutorials and *asynchronous* reflective activities, such as the use of e-mail. It is intended, however, to eventually explore the educational potential offered by other telematic-assisted learning systems, such as satellite broadcast television.

This project has attempted to find solutions towards two key problems affecting higher education needs in the southwest UK region, these being:

1. greater accessibility to higher education professional development opportunities for life-long learning students who are otherwise disadvantaged through geographic isolation, full-time employment pressures, family and other social commitments; and,

2. an increase in participation rates for professional skills updating through distance education, in order to create a better-educated and more flexible workforce.

The project, therefore, impacted upon a clear set of regional social needs, satisfying the common aspirations of both the EU RATIO initiative and the university's higher education focus. This telematic-based distance education solution envisaged developing a balance between the university's learning resources available over the Internet and live-audience interactive learning experiences through RATIO and other videoconference centres across the UK southwest region.

The identification, development and testing of a Web page authoring kit, suitable for practical university staff development, represented an original contribution. It also achieved viable solutions to some of the Information and Learning Technology (ILT) issues highlighted in the UK government's Higginson (Further Education Funding Council, 1999) report, regarding the difficulties of getting staff to implement flexible distance education through information technology learning curricula and superhighway learning resources. Indeed, the report recommends that priority be given to learning materials development and that proper arrangements are made to provide staff with support, information, and advice in all ILT areas of development, including solving the funding issues arising from delivering pedagogy in this manner. These ILT implementation and delivery issues have also been recognized in the European Union's white paper on education and training, leading to the funding of a wide range of telematic-assisted learning applied research projects (European Union, 1995). The UK government's Dearing Report (1997) into higher education also considers the importance that information and communication technologies will play in widening access opportunities. The Times Higher Education Supplement (THES) (1997) summarized a key recognition from Dearing that "Over the next ten years the delivery of some course materials and much of the organization and communication of course arrangements will be conducted by computer" (p. 1). However, the THES also reports Dearing's cautions for the proper management of such learning technologies and cites the need for "educational intervention and support structures [that are] sensitive to the needs and practices of lecturers and students [and asks] how educational technologies can be most effectively deployed" (p. 1). This implies the need for university online course designers and planners to identify the instructional pedagogic and technical protocols involved in delivering quality higher education programs in this particular format and learning style.

This project was a small, but important, part of the EU's overall telematic program. Our purpose was to experiment with our telematic-assisted distance learning module throughout the southwest UK RATIO economic development region and determine a pedagogic model of good practice for future expansion both nationally and internationally. Information and communications technology media resources, such as the Internet, have allowed for such a vision to take place. However, the pedagogic communications patterns for collaborative telelearning constitute a radically different educational delivery process when compared to conventional learning systems (Aviv & Golan, 1998). The existing masters delivery model offered by the university had already attracted a large number of students and this new distance education program was considered to be one way of providing additional recruitment opportunities. This project has, therefore, explored one solution towards solving an access problem that often prevents expansion in higher education owing to both financial and geographical constraints. An appropriate policy that can overcome these problems and enable the flexible delivery of higher education distance learning was thought to provide one way of optimizing the university's organization of human and financial resources. Success in telematic-assisted distance learning potentially offers a new delivery extension to the integrated masters program, leading to a wider and more diverse range of courses.

The specific aims of the project were:

1. To develop a university Internet Web site facility, capable of delivering flexible masters courses via this telematic platform.
2. To pilot and determine the pedagogic processes and necessary support requirements underpinning the conversion of the module "IT for Personal Development and Project Management" into such a flexible distance learning package.
3. To develop flexible distance learning synchronous IT communications solutions for seminars, tutorials, etc., through RATIO videoconference centers across the region.
4. To evaluate the effectiveness of the flexible online distance learning solutions developed in terms of key findings gleaned from involved staff and distance education participants, and, further, to identify the significant lessons learned with consequent implications for teaching and learning in higher education.

THE IMPLEMENTATION OF THE PROJECT

The development activity associated with the preparation and production of an online distance learning module is not the key focus of this article, however, the need for a clear staff development support process for all intending remote tutors was identified. The pedagogic protocols listed in Table 1 suggest the process a tutor may follow in converting conventional higher education course modules into a new telematic-assisted distance learning format and explain the type of technical and academic support services required. However, the main focus of this article is to concentrate on the pedagogic implications of actually implementing a remote learning online module, rather than those of designing it, which was earlier reported by Rodd and Coombs (1997). The

TABLE 1. Executive Summary of Key Pedagogic Recommendations

Pedagogic area identified	Pedagogic protocols suggested
Authoring a remote learning curriculum. Need for a staff development support process for all remote tutors operating as curriculum authors. The pedagogic protocols listed opposite suggest the process a tutor may follow and the type of technical and academic support services required. Essentially, a courseware development support service is required for remote learning tutors. The tutor also needs to possess a wide range of generic IT application area skills, e.g., word-processing, DTP design and layout skills and knowledge of multimedia-type instructional systems.	• Preparatory phase of collating all course documentation into a Web-ready file format • Curriculum reappraisal. Identifying prior learning requirements, core learning elements and principle content. • Use of 'storyboard' templates as a mapping tool to establish key educational hyperlinks. • Academic linked references to external Web sites related to the course module. • Use of Web-based discussion group facilities beyond e-mail, i.e., bulletin board and chat room.
Webministration–technical and administrative support service. This project identified the need for a suitable technical and administrative system, which supports online learning. In particular, the perceived Webministration services would include the protocols listed opposite.	• Web-based course registration services. • Internet e-mail access by remote learners to administrative & academic staff for essential troubleshooting-type queries. • A Web master technical backup and consultancy service.
Improving remote learning academic participation. The need for a virtual faculty to support remote learners was identified. This includes Webministration support services, listed above, as well as additional telematic resources that are summarized in the technical and pedagogic communications protocols opposite.	• A tutor-independent online service, with the aim of providing consistent information and better access to faculty resources. • The need for appropriately archived video courseware material. • The need for a cheaper and easily accessible multipoint desktop videoconference system over the Wideband Internet. • The need for a user-friendly Web-conferencing facility that will enable online social interaction.

delivery process of this module is described in the following three stages:

1. Recruitment of participants
2. Delivery of the module
3. Evaluation of student and tutor experiences

Recruitment of Participants

Prospective students were invited to attend an introduction and induction evening prior to accessing the module. At this event the course tutors and administrative staff were available to: explain the process of delivering, assessing and evaluating the module; discuss any student concerns; assess accessibility and compatibility of the hardware and prospective venue that students intended to use in studying the module; and, identify and discuss students' expectations about–and potential obstacles to–successful completion of the module.

Twenty students attended the introduction and induction evening, from which 16 people were enrolled. All the students had appropriate entry qualifications for enrollment in the integrated masters program and were adults who either were involved in, or had previously worked in, education, training and related fields. Difficulties in obtaining access to suitable IT hardware and viable venue sites were the reasons given for the four people who did not enroll. This technological access reason proved to be a common significant factor in later course dropouts.

During the induction session the 16 students were asked to complete a short questionnaire to identify previous IT experience, in order to ascertain the likely needs and level of IT support during the module.

Delivery of the Module

Once enrolled, the 16 students were provided with the module's Web site address (see Figure 1), user name and password to access the seven learning sessions (see Figure 2).

The module was authored so as to allow general public access to some information, but with the key learning sessions and tutor e-mail access protected by a user name and password. Students were asked to signal their participation in the content of the module by submitting an introductory e-mail about themselves for their tutors and peers. Students were then asked to respond to the tutor's e-mail requesting details about their project assignment. An e-mail distribution list was set up to

FIGURE 1. Main Activities Menu for IMP Distance Education Module

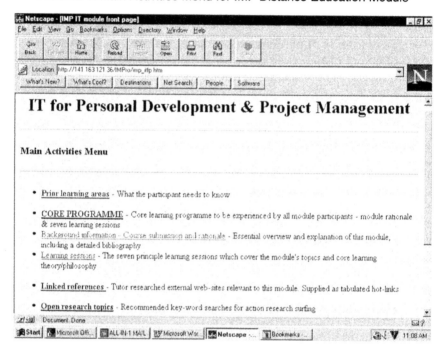

facilitate communication between tutors and students. Students were then required to access and complete the learning sessions in their preferred venue at their own time and pace. The tutors encouraged students to communicate about on-the-job difficulties encountered during the module and distributed e-mail responses to frequently asked questions (FAQs) for all group members. Students were also encouraged to communicate with fellow peers about their experiences encountered while undertaking the module, thereby encouraging the establishment of a support group. The learning sessions needed to be completed in sufficient time for students to prepare and submit an appropriate project assignment by a set date. At least one videoconference session was planned during the delivery of the module. Numerous problems related to the delivery of the module subsequently emerged.

Evaluation of Student and Tutor Experience

Project evaluation was carried out through qualitative analysis of the following pedagogic domains:

FIGURE 2. The Core Learning Sessions

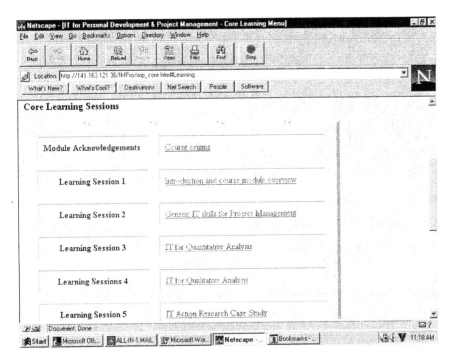

1. Ease and support issues related to developing a flexible distance learning telematics package by remotely located university staff.
2. Extent to which the pedagogic aim of the masters module was actually achieved through flexible distance learning assessment methods.
3. Student attitudes regarding both participation and learning through a flexible distance learning delivery format. Interviews, both personal and e-mail, coupled with post-module evaluation feedback reports were deployed.
4. Tutor experience of, and attitudes to, teaching and delivering a module in this particular format via chronological recording of key on-the-job personal learning events.

Conversational learning encounters between tutors, students and fellow students enrolled in the module were made available through built-in Internet e-mail facilities offered through the Web site. Conventional telecommunication support services were offered as a back-up facility, that is, the use of telephone contact numbers, fax, etc. In practice, however, these services were rarely employed.

RESEARCH FINDINGS

Action research data was collected and evaluated on four areas:

1. Student attrition
2. Previous experience in using IT
3. E-mail correspondence
4. Personal reflections of the tutor.

Student Attrition

Student attrition was a major issue in the delivery of this distance learning module. In the four weeks following the introduction and induction evening, eight of the enrolled students withdrew from the module. The two main reasons cited were a lack of accessibility to suitable hardware, and the participant's employment pressures. The project was dependent upon the operation of RATIO centres throughout the southwest of England. The delivery and installation of IT equipment to access the Internet and to participate in videoconferences ran well behind schedule, which meant that none of the RATIO centres could be fully used by the students. The remaining students had to find alternative venues. This task proved extremely difficult and resulted in the loss of another five students. Pressure from employment proved to be another factor in student attrition. A majority of the students worked as trainers in higher education UK colleges. These sectors were, and are, experiencing major structural upheaval, which resulted in the loss of an additional three students who were obliged to take on extra workload responsibilities in order to retain their jobs. These students would have withdrawn from the module regardless of its mode of delivery, and this highlights the impact of employment pressures on adult students.

Over the following four weeks another four students withdrew. Two students considered that their low level of competence with IT would result in their inability to successfully complete the module. One student, who suffered from multiple disabilities, withdrew because the university was unable to meet specific educational needs for a voice-activated computer. The final student withdrew because he was returning early to his home in Cyprus.

The remaining group of four students progressed through the learning sessions over a period of approximately four months. However, of these, only two students completed the module requirement of submitting and passing a work-based action research project assignment. While the other two students had completed the technical requirements of the learning sessions, they failed to submit the rigorous post-graduate project assignment.

Survey of Previous Experience With IT

The original 16 students who enrolled on the module completed a short one-page questionnaire that aimed to identify their previous experience with the type of IT skills on which the module was based. The results are summarized in Table 2.

The majority of students reported previous experience of using word-processors, with approximately half of them having prior experience of e-mail and the Internet. The majority of students had not participated in videoconferencing.

In relation to the type of system that the students intended to use, 12 indicated that they would use a standard PC, three would use a Macintosh, and one would use both systems.

Although the workplace and home were specified by the students as venues where they would be most likely to access the module, 11 indicated that they would probably use both places in order to more fully participate. Given that the RATIO centres were not fully operational during the module, two students had to find other suitable venues. (See Table 3.)

Finally, the students were asked to rate themselves in terms of their level of confidence for using IT on a four-point scale (very confident, confident, unconfident, very unconfident). Half of the students (8) reported that they felt "confident," seven reported feeling "unconfident," and one student reported feeling "very confident" in using IT. Interestingly, only two students withdrew because of feelings of incompetence with using IT. The data obtained suggested that adult student attrition was mainly associated with social factors unrelated to any lack of confidence in using IT.

Qualitative Analysis of E-Mail Correspondence

E-mail correspondence (and just four telephone calls) generally connected to technical and academic-related problems. Initial technical problems were related to obtaining the correct URL address for accessing the module Web site on the Internet, and incorrect, or changed,

TABLE 2. Experience with Different Information Technologies

IT application area	Yes	No
Word-processing	15	1
E-mail	7	9
The Internet	9	7
Videoconferencing	1	15

TABLE 3. Choice of Venue for Accessing the Module

Type of venue	Number of students
Home	4
Work	8
University campus	2
RATIO center	2

e-mail addresses. Unfortunately, following the introduction and induction evening–when the module's Web site address on the Internet was provided to students–it was subsequently decided by the university's technical support staff to change this address. Although inserting the new address into the home page rectified this problem, it nevertheless resulted in considerable student confusion. The change of address was followed almost immediately by the university's computer system "going down" for a couple of days, a likely situation that the students had not been forewarned about, thus undermining their confidence and increasing their sense of social isolation (Aviv & Golan, 1998). In setting up the module on the Internet, technical staff from two university departments had been involved. It is important that only one department (or agency) be responsible for frequent communications to all systems-users. Coombs (1997) identified this as an essential "Webministration" facility that underpins the technical and administrative support services of any remote learning virtual faculty.

Owing to a lack of any central Webministration service, distance learner users were supplied with incorrect e-mail addresses and weren't sufficiently informed of any vital system changes. In the early stage of the module's delivery, one of the tutors took a position in another country, also resulting in a change of e-mail address. Some students, who had a limited understanding about the precise nature of e-mail addresses, provided inaccurate contact details. One student changed her e-mail address during the module and then provided inaccurate contact details. Consequently, the distribution lists became incorrect at frequent intervals, resulting in students not receiving replies to e-mail or e-mailed correspondence. After these initial technical problems were overcome the student group had decreased to four. For this remaining group the type of technical query changed from simple problems–as described above–to a set of more complex IT user problems. These included the encoding and decoding of e-mail attachments between incompatible non-standard e-mail software systems; how to access the Integrated Masters Program and other academic-related Web sites; creating and saving of graphics as GIF files and word-processed material, so that they can be sent as split text and graphics files as e-mail attachments; and, finally, pedagogic queries related to setting up and preparing for a videoconference seminar session.

All of these problems were resolved by the remote academic support tutor through the e-mail contact system. This unforeseen IT user support service added considerably to the tutor's burden–contributing to the large 73 online contact hours that were recorded and reported by the tutor. This is compared to the conventional delivery of the same module, which was previously delivered in only 30 hours of contact time. These additional hours were divided between the identified three roles of technical, administrative, and academic support services. Clearly, it is essential that students have immediate access to technical and administrative support services for such a technology-dependent learning system. However, it is recommended that these two roles should be provided by a centralized tutor-independent Webministration service, with academic module support residing with the tutor. This under-estimation of the essential virtual support services required to effectively deliver and manage a distance learning higher education module has been recognized by Gawith (1998). Gawith maintains that the real costs of telelearning: "... involves not only the direct costs of the telecommunications hardware, software and usage charges, but indirect costs that are, arguably, ultimately more significant" (p. 5). Gawith defines these indirect costs in terms of familiarization time for the teachers to learn how to integrate the technology into their curriculum. This would include the time required to rethink and redesign these programs into the new delivery formats required. Hence, in order to deliver the same [sic!] masters course, the tutor spent two working days per week over a four-month period engaged in this instructional redesigning task alone. Other hidden costs include ensuring that the participants have sufficient technology and information skills required to attempt the telematic learning tasks. Gawith also acknowledges that telelearning requires more time than conventionally delivered courses for the monitoring and guiding of student learning, as we found to be the case for distance delivery of an integrated masters program module.

Because of tutor unavailability due to holiday periods and absences related to other academic duties, some students reported concern about delays in responses to e-mailed correspondence. Tutors also found they could not always contact students, which created uncertainty about their continued participation in the module. It is important that all participants alert group members if they are going to be offline for any significant period of time. An unexplained offline period of absence creates a kind of *cybervoid*. This is a communications vacuum that engenders a feeling of anxiety among the rest of the participants in the group. Aviv and Golan (1998) recognize this as a negative effect upon the remote learning process and suggest avoiding it by instigating a pedagogic communications protocol that includes a combination of personal support learning services and mutual activities with other participants in the form of collaborative group work projects. Indeed, Suler (1997) recommends that in order to make virtual learning communities work, a clear set of learning principles needs to be established. Suler's set of pedagogic and social cyber-protocols includes:

1. Use software that promotes good discussions.
2. Don't impose a length limitation on postings.
3. Front-load your system with talkative, diverse people.
4. Let the users resolve their own disputes.
5. Provide institutional memory.
6. Promote continuity.
7. Be host to a particular interest group.
8. Provide places for children.
9. Confront the users with a crisis.

A transparent socio-pedagogic communications protocol linked to Webministration administrative and technical support services, tutor academic support, and other distant learner participants are therefore a recommended essential infrastructure for any expansion to this service. Trentin (2000), who suggests that online education systems represent a third generation distance education, also supports this idea. He links the technology with user interactivity and program quality, suggesting that there is "a strict link between quality and the capability to manage a learning process based on the active participation of all its beneficiaries" (p. 18).

A range of academic queries was raised in student e-mail correspondence. These related mainly to: (a) definitions of academic terminology, (b) requests for feedback on student work; (c) questions about theoretical and methodological issues; (d) requests for traditional printed resource materials; (e) a request for information about administrative and library matters; and (f) the use and value of reflection in academic work and other matters directly related to the scholastic content of the module. Where appropriate, the tutor's reply was distributed to all of the group members, as were all relevant suggestions and comments from the students.

Although the students could have performed traditional written end-of-module evaluations, the small number of students made this process redundant. Instead, the two students, who successfully completed all seven learning sessions and had submitted an appropriate project assignment, were contacted personally to discuss their experiences about the strengths and weaknesses of online distance learning. The consensus was that there was more time and work associated with undertaking a module in this format than in traditional delivery modes, which corresponds with Gawith's (1998) findings discussed earlier. While the students thought that they had learned a lot, they described some of the theoretical online reading as "heavy going." The students thought that two competing demands were made on them. First, the demand of learning advanced IT skills that enabled them to undertake the distance learning module; and, second, the demand of learning related to academic content requirements.

The students recognized that there were initial "teething problems" associated with the technical aspects of the module, but acknowledged that these were overcome through the regular e-mail and encouraging personal support offered by the tutors. The lack of face-to-face social interaction with the rest of the group was considered to be a disadvantage. It was understood that this aspect could have been overcome with a more appropriate videoconferencing solution, such as the system suggested by Sharpe, Coombs, and Gopinathan (1999), who encourage the use of user-friendly and low-cost multipoint desktop videoconferencing (MDVC) equipment on a broadband Internet service. Only one videoconference session was organized, in which only one of the students could participate at the university's venue due to technical and time difficulties. The other student linked-up separately via her school's videoconference resource, but all three venues could only communicate via point-to-point. A multi-point bridge-server was not available between the three venues, so three-way communication was stymied. The tutors also recognized that some of the students' problems with the module were associated with their inexperience in authoring appropriately formatted graphics and text files and sending them via e-mail. These technical problems are likely to be resolved in future online distance learning packages.

Personal Reflections of the Tutor

The remote tutor identified and recorded a wide range of problems and successes associated with the online delivery of this module. The key pedagogic issues identified were as follows:

1. The lack of a distance learning systems protocol that delineates open support between the three core user areas: online administration services, IT technical services, and academic services. These duties were unanticipated and left to the online module tutor to sort out.
2. The lack of any user-friendly videoconference facility that could easily connect the tutor and the group together for multi-point private conversations, i.e., a technical solution is required along with appropriate *synchronous pedagogic communications protocols* governing its use.
3. The need for a clear Web-based "netiquette" and online protocol from which both distance learners and module tutors can overcome the problems of remoteness and lack of face-to-face contact, i.e., *asynchronous pedagogic communications protocols* are required.
4. While the student attrition dropout from the module was high, the quality of the completed projects was excellent and fully met the integrated masters program standards, thereby accrediting community-based action research projects via a university online distance learning program.

From these cautionary experiences the tutor has recommended the following pedagogic and technical communications protocols for all future online masters courses:

1. The creation of a Webministration service to centrally coordinate the distance learning support service. That is, both a centralized forum

and intermediary service through which the Masters online modules may be administered. The service would include online registrations, dissemination of necessary regulations and user-contact time-credit protocols, and assistance with IT technical problems. The Webministration coordinating facility would form the academic support infrastructure of an online virtual faculty and could offer global access to the UK masters program (see Table 3 for more details).

2. The studio-based videoconference facility offered by providers such as PictureTel© Corporation are considered to be inappropriate and inflexible to the distance learner's needs for an easy-access face-to-face solution. Instead, the tutor has recommended a multipoint desktop videoconference solution, such as is being currently offered by the joint research initiative between Cornell University and the CU-SeeMe© Corporation and adopted by Sharpe, Coombs and Gopinathan (1999). This system offers server space for "bridging" multi-point desktop video-conference sessions via the client-users' own PC on the Internet. They currently offer an education and business users service. The education service offers videoconference access through their NASA-sponsored Global Schools Network (GSN) initiative. The business service, which includes many university clients, offers paid server access or the possibility for clients to run their own Unix©-based server with the desktop software that runs on both the Windows© 95/98 PC and Macintosh© operating systems. It also offers H.323 international standards compatibility, meaning that desktop multi-point videoconferencing can occur with other systems, i.e., Wideband CU-SeeMe© internet solutions communicating with PictureTel's© ISDN systems.

OUTCOMES AND DISCUSSION

Several key benefits and outcomes stemmed from this project and included the following:

1. The development and running of a dedicated Web site, which included full interactive student participatory features, such as Internet e-mail, which responded to the mainly asynchronous communications needs and demands of the learners and tutors.
2. The conversion and testing of an existing university masters course module into a suitable flexible distance learning online format.

3. The identification and development of a suitable Web-based editor, which was capable of being used as a staff development authoring tool by the concerned faculty member.
4. The piloting of videoconference resources as a means of satisfying the perceived face-to-face synchronous communications requirements underpinning online delivery of a higher education program.
5. The development of a suitable format with regards to the assessment and evaluation of flexible distance learning online programs.
6. The involvement of current masters' students in using advanced information technology skills associated with technology-assisted flexible distance learning programs.
7. A demonstration of applying telematic systems to the delivery of higher education programs.

Although the final group of students was small, the quality of their submitted responses to the seven learning sessions and assignments demonstrated that the project had a significant impact on the quality of learning. The most important quality-related issue is that of improved student access to postgraduate professional training programs. The students who completed the module would not have enrolled in a traditional delivery mode because of various social commitments. Higher education learning opportunities were therefore realized through the medium of a telematic-assisted flexible distance learning program, offered in a geographically sparsely populated region of the UK.

An important impact on the quality of learning was the creation of a flexible distance learning medium, which promoted the ethos of student autonomy with regards to their own learning. This pedagogic concept underpins the aims of effective adult learning and satisfies the deep learning criteria of the masters program. It also fulfills Trentin's (2000) notion that student empowerment in the form of active engagement in the online medium's process is a measure of its pedagogic quality. Good quality telematic-assisted learning programs, with proper higher education accredited status, can achieve Boud's (1981) vision of developing the educational qualities and personal skills that underpin the successful performance and capability of the autonomous learner. This is further underpinned by Harri-Augstein and Thomas' (1991) notion of the self-organized learner, whereby an individual's learning capabilities can be enhanced through technology assistants that they refer to as an intelligent learning system. Coombs (1995) further elaborates this notion of an intelligent learning system in terms of a knowledge elicitation system, whereby information technology-assisted learning is considered in terms of its interactive learning capability with an individual learner. It is therefore understood that the quality of learner-learning with an information technology software system can be explained in terms of the learners being able to systematically manage their own elicitations in the form of self-organized reflective construing experiences. From this perspective, knowledge is considered as being relative to the user, as learner, via focused information technology-assisted reflections, construed and elicited by the person in the form of meaningful learning conversations. This form of internal knowledge construction from self-managed reflective experiences represents a new learning theory that Coombs and Smith (1998) refer to as "conversational constructivism." They maintain that:

> IT tools used for activities which encourage, stimulate and focus meaningful reflection can be viewed as knowledge modeling devices that facilitate learning in a social context. This particular paradigm empowers *learner control* of the *learning process* using appropriate conversational tools to achieve one's learning goals and provides a valid learning theory that explains the motivational role and educational value of a conversational learning environment. (p. 27)

Given this understanding of how information technology/telematic learning systems may impact upon the personal learning capability of the learner–coupled with the demands of higher education, such as developing the learners' reflective skills–it can easily be seen how appropriately designed learning technologies could bring considerable benefits to outreach members of the community participating in a distance education scheme.

Additionally, the personal involvement of the tutor in developing his/her curriculum through an action research project is supported by educational critical thinkers like Stenhouse (1975) and Elliot (1991) who support the notion of teacher as experimenter of his or her curriculum. Evaluation of the ongoing curriculum development experiences of the tutor involved in converting a module into a flexible distance learning format was a valuable staff development exercise. An action research reflective learning biography was kept as a means of project management review and self-evaluation of the important lessons learned as they were experienced on-the-job.

The module chosen as a pilot for this project offered a diverse curriculum range, which embodied the spirit of the central masters program tasks and its deep criteria, while lending itself towards the use of technology-assisted reflective tools. Clearly, the telematic media adopted, that is, Internet Webpages and PictureTel© videoconference facilities, lent themselves to the central IT ethos of the module itself. This enabled participants to critically appraise advanced information technology-assisted learning systems in terms of their ability to operate them successfully as knowledge elicitation systems. A central axiom of the module "IT for Personal Development and Project Management" critically appraises IT in terms of its ability to be used as a conversational learning tool that can be employed as a means of personal development. These IT reflective-tools assist participants to carry out a small-scale action research project from within their own social and working environment (Coombs, 1997). This masters program design issue was raised in the United States, with Tom (1999) reporting that, "Teachers dislike these (educational masters) programs. They view them as detached from the daily practice of schooling" (p. 245). This suggests the potential merit in implementing a flexible online Master of Education program that addresses professional teacher development needs through accreditation of action research curriculum projects.

Information technology project management techniques for this community-based online masters course included the use of:

1. The Internet to research contemporary background information of a participant's subject/professional development field.
2. E-mail as an asynchronous critical thinking communications medium to share research questions and concerns with project supervisors and other team members.
3. Spreadsheets for quantitative data analysis and graphical presentation.
4. Word-processing facilities to keep a computerized reflective log/account of key project events and submit the final assessment dissertation.

A key part of this masters module required one-to-one synchronous tutorials to negotiate the participant's work-based project and discuss individual needs and assessment methods best suited to achieving the assessment task. Videoconferencing provided a means of giving this kind of support to distance learners, but in practice proved to be impossible to implement owing to the unwieldy nature of existing studio-based videoconference solutions. However, the PictureTel© ISDN system employed did provide the bonus of sharing an IT task with a distance learner, despite the difficulty of arranging prior access and use. Clearly, it is now possible to conduct interactive synchronous IT software demonstrations and exercises. This IT module involved the conventional use and tutor demonstration of Excel© and SPSS©, which could have been achieved remotely online through a more user-friendly multipoint desktop videoconference system that has an IT task-sharing management facility for interactive participation.

Difficulties Encountered

A number of obstacles to the development and delivery of the module were encountered by the tutor and students. For the tutor, a lack of support in the administrative, library, and technical areas; inadequate time allocation and resources for the development of the module; and, recognition by the university administration of the needs of a remote and/or home tutor were all identified. For students, the major obstacle was accessing equipment to undertake the module tasks. Contrary to expectation, the RATIO centres were not fully resourced with the equipment necessary for students to undertake the module during the trial period. In addition, a student with multiple disabilities was unable to gain access to equipment that would have allowed participation in the module. Where alternative venues were identified, such as colleges, schools or home systems, the capacity of these systems could not always handle the demands of the technology. Some students found that the challenge of mastering the technology was far greater than expected and felt that they could not handle both the technology and content together. However, most students reported that the major advantage of this module was the opportunity of working in their chosen venue, in their own time, and at their own pace.

CONCLUSION

The key benefits of this project will impact upon those participating students, drawn principally from the southwest of England, who wish to pursue professional development in higher education. Another key benefit is the staff development of all those involved in this project, including the participating project team, through their personal experiences of innovative practice that have led to new pedagogical knowledge and skills of how to deliver masters modules through remote learning technologies. As a consequence of cross-institutional collaborative involvement, the RATIO partner institutions will clearly benefit in the future through the perceived enhancement of their reputation as leaders in delivering distance education, despite the setbacks reported in this project. Table 1 summarizes the executive recommendations made regarding the technical and pedagogic support protocols required for delivering higher education by telematic-assisted distance education. Indeed, Barnard (1997) recognizes the potential to create virtual universities through the combination of Web-based courses with other media technologies, such as satellite TV, CD-ROM and other video-based avenues. However, Barnard cautions us with some examples of how bad online instructional design of courses has led to poor implementation, with staff concerns and resistance to adopt these new pedagogic practices owing to ill thought-out consequences such as additional workloads. He cites the unfortunate example of a colleague who has to spend between four and five hours per day reading and responding to e-mail from a class of 50 online students where, clearly, an asynchronous communications pedagogic protocol affecting this kind of course delivery issue is severely lacking.

The recommendations made in Table 1 attempt to recognize the pedagogic areas affected by setting up a virtual learning faculty for higher education and fully agree with the changing pedagogic roles recommended for ILT tutors in the Further Education Funding Councils (1999) report "Networking Lifelong Learning." They recognize that:

> the role of the tutor will be transformed to that of a learning coach [with] changing work patterns relating to location, weekly and annual timetable, and learner caseload. The core competencies required for learners, and in which the tutor or coach must specialize, include (as well as conventional core skills): learning methodology; project management; information analysis and dissemination; problem solving; and, design and presentation. (p. 20)

In addition to the valuable lessons learned and pedagogic recommendations made by this project, we can see that the future educational profession has much to gain from the new insights and transferability of ideas from this distance learning project. Clearly, it has made an original contribution toward the greater understanding of Web-based pedagogy, impacting upon the management, theory, and practice of teaching and learning in higher education.

REFERENCES

Aviv, R., & Golan, G. (1998). Pedagogic communication patterns in collaborative telelearning. *Journal of Educational Technology Systems, 26*(3), 201-208.

Barnard, J. (1997). The World Wide Web and higher education: The promise of virtual universities and online libraries. *Educational Technology, 37*(3), 30-35.

Boud, D. (1981). *Developing student autonomy in learning.* London: Kogan Page.

Coombs, S. (1995). *Design and conversational evaluation of an IT learning environment based on self-organized learning.* Unpublished doctoral thesis. London, England: Brunel University.

Coombs, S. (1997). Applied telematics for interdisciplinary action research. In Chen Lai Keat & Toh Kok Aun (Eds.), *Research across the disciplines*, Proceedings of the Singapore Educational Research Association. Singapore: National Institute of Education.

Coombs, S., & Smith, I. (1998). Designing a self-organized conversational learning environment. *Educational Technology, 38*(3), 17-28.

Dearing, R. (1997). *National committee of inquiry into higher education.* The Dearing Report. London: HMSO. [Online]. Available: *http://www.leeds.ac.uk/educol/ncihe/*

Elliot, J. (1991). *Action research for educational change.* Milton Keynes: Open University Press.

European Union (1995). *Teaching and learning–towards the learning society.* Directive 12 (DGXII), the European Union's White Paper on education and training. [Online]. Available: *http://www.europa.eu.int/en/comm/dg22/lbhp.html*

Further Education Funding Council (FEFC) (1999). *Networking lifelong learning: An Information and Learning Technology development strategy for further education.* A consultation report prepared by the Further Education Information and Learning Technology Committee. FEFC publication, UK. [Online]. Available: *http://194. 66.249.219/documents/othercouncilpublications/other_pdf/9918suppl.pdf*

Gawith, G. (1998). The real cost of telelearning: A case study. *Computers in NZ Schools*, March, 5-14.

Harri-Augstein, S., & Thomas, L. (1991). *Learning conversations.* London: Routledge.

Rodd, J., & Coombs, S. (1997). Development and evaluation of an experimental Integrated Masters Program Web site as part of a flexible and distance education learning policy for the University of Plymouth. CD-ROM proceedings paper no. 182–CAL'97, University of Exeter, March 1997. [Online]. Available: *http://www. media.uwe.ac.uk/~masoud/cal-7/papers/rodd.htm*

Sharpe, L., Coombs, S., & Gopinathan, S. (1999). Computer communications discourse for Singapore's practicum students. In Margit Waas (Ed.), *Enhancing learning: Challenge of integrating thinking and information technology into the curriculum*, Vol. 1 & 2, Ch. 2: Information technology, 216-222. Singapore: National Institute of Education.

Stenhouse, L. (1975). *An introduction to curriculum research and development.* London: Heinemann.

Suler, J. (1997). *Making virtual communities work.* Rider University. [Online]. Available: *http://www.rider.edu/users/suler/psycyber/commwork.html*

Times Higher Education Supplement (THES) (1997). Dearing & IT multimedia special feature: page 1, No. 39, August 1, 1997.

Tom, A. (1999). Reinventing master's degree study for experienced teachers. *Journal of Teacher Education, 50*(4), 245-254.

Trentin, G. (2000). The quality-interactivity relationship in distance education. *Educational Technology, 40*(1), 17-27.

OTHER WEB SITE REFERENCES

The Integrated Masters Program (IMP) Web site: University of Plymouth, UK. [Online]. Available: *http://www.fae.plym.ac.uk/postgrad/imp.html*

The White Pine CU-SeeMe Web site for Web-based multipoint desktop videoconferencing (MDVC) software solutions. [Online]. Available: *http://www.wpine.com/*

Lorraine Sherry

Internet and World Wide Web Usage in an Institution of Higher Learning

SUMMARY. This paper reports the results of a five-year case study of the use of online tools: Internet, e-mail, and the WWW in a Graduate School of Education at an urban university located on a commuter campus. The conceptual framework was independently developed, but because of the striking parallel with activity theory, activity theory became the overall framework for interpreting findings. Ten research questions were investigated using a survey repeated in 1995 and 1997; interviews of faculty, staff, and students; a focus group; and an analysis of electronic artifacts. There were four principal findings. Self-efficacy × perceived value persisted across time and across programs as success facilitators. Personal/cultural compatibility, rather than time, separated earlier from later adopters. "Finding a voice and having something to say," a factor identified under various names by other researchers, posed a challenge for students and faculty alike. Users valued personal scaffolding but had individual preferences concerning specific types of scaffolding. The study resulted in a set of recommendations, some of which have now been implemented. *[Article copies available for a fee from The Haworth Document Delivery Service: 1-800-342-9678. E-mail address: <getinfo@haworthpressinc.com> Website: <http://www.HaworthPress.com> © 2001 by The Haworth Press, Inc. All rights reserved.]*

LORRAINE SHERRY is Research Associate, RMC Research Corporation, Writer Square, Suite 540, 1512 Larimer Street, Denver, CO 80202 (E-mail: sherry@rmcdenver.com).

[Haworth co-indexing entry note]: "Internet and World Wide Web Usage in an Institution of Higher Learning." Sherry, Lorraine. Co-published simultaneously in *Computers in the Schools* (The Haworth Press, Inc.) Vol. 17, No. 3/4. 2001, pp. 91-105; and: *The Web in Higher Education: Assessing the Impact and Fulfilling the Potential* (ed: Cleborne D. Maddux, and D. LaMont Johnson) The Haworth Press, Inc., 2001, pp. 91-105. Single or multiple copies of this article are available for a fee from The Haworth Document Delivery Service [1-800-342-9678, 9:00 a.m. - 5:00 p.m. (EST). E-mail address: getinfo@haworthpressinc.com].

91

KEYWORDS. Internet, e-mail, World Wide Web, WWW, self-efficacy, personal scaffolding, diffusion

This investigation began in the fall of 1994, when the director of the Instructional Technology (I.T.) doctoral program at an urban graduate school of education and an ad hoc group of graduate students formed the Internet Task Force to explore "Internet tool" usage within the Division of Technology and Special Services. At that time, this division housed the I.T. doctoral and master's programs. The group focused on exploring the use of Internet tools to support teaching and learning, rather than acquiring a set of technology skills for its own sake. In this context, Internet tools were defined as e-mail, a FirstClass™ electronic conferencing system (known as CEO), and the World Wide Web (WWW). The Internet Task Force had a fourfold purpose: (a) to enable members of the I.T. doctoral and master's programs to join the Internet culture; (b) to develop a knowledge-building environment for graduate classes and seminars; (c) to conduct research on technology adoption and develop a set of recommendations based on facilitators that they identified; and (d) to provide support for new telecommunications users.

A key point in Soviet psychology, attributed to Vygotsky, is the emphasis on the use of tools in the development of human mental processes. "The tool is not simply added on to human activity; rather, it transforms it" (Tikhomirov, 1981, p. 270). Engestrom expands Vygotsky's notion to conceptualize human activity as an interdependent system that ties the individual to a larger cultural context. In Engestrom's (1996, 1998) conceptual framework, known as Activity Theory, the activities in which an individual engages tend to connect six elements, namely: (a) the individual subject or actor, (b) the object of action together with an intentional outcome, (c) the tools or instruments used to carry out the activity, (d) the community of which the subject is a part, (e) the norms and conventions of use of those tools, and (f) the division of labor that characterizes individual actions within local collaborative activities. These elements–tools, rules, roles, and relationships–are all interrelated. Changing one will invariably affect the rest of the system.

Over a four-year period, the task force published several papers that documented the results of their surveys, interviews, focus groups, and observations concerning Internet tool use within the Division of Technology and Special Services (Wilson, Lowry, Koneman, & Osman-Jouchoux, 1994; Ryder & Wilson, 1996; Sherry & the Internet Task Force, 1996; Wilson, Ryder, McCahan, & Sherry, 1996; Sherry, 1997; Sherry & Myers, 1998). The initial survey, conducted in 1995, was limited to the Division of Special Services. It was repeated in 1997 to include the entire Graduate School of Education. The case study described here (Sherry, 1998) used mixed methods to investigate the factors that affected the use of the Internet within the Graduate School of Education as a whole.

INTERPRETIVE FRAMEWORK

This case study combined both empirical research within the graduate school and an extensive review of relevant literature to identify 28 distinct factors that affect Internet diffusion. To summarize, the process of change and diffusion begins with individuals' characteristics and perceptions, coupled with the cultural norms and legitimate activities of the learning community of which they are a part. It progresses through various processes of dealing with the design of the innovation, learning how to use its associated tools, utilizing the communication channels of the organization, and making effective use of both the impersonal and personal support structure of the organization. Finally, it ends with cognitive restructuring and transformation of perspectives among those individuals and the learning groups of which they are a part. This may lead to reaffirmation of the adoption decision, with the adopter influencing other colleagues and students to adopt it, or it may lead to the reluctant use or outright rejection of the innovation.

Using this process model as an organizing framework, the 28 factors identified in the literature review and associated empirical research were grouped into six clusters. (See Figure 1.) These clusters were used as a starting point for formulating a new model of Internet diffusion by institutions of higher education.

The clusters of factors in Figure 1 can be compared with the six elements of an activity system (Engestrom, 1998), as shown in Table 1. Because of this close similarity between the two models, Activity Theory was used as the interpretive framework for the current study.

METHOD

Preliminary Investigations

In spring 1995, three important activities took place. A member of the Internet Task Force interviewed representative members of the I.T.

FIGURE 1. Clusters of Factors that Affect Internet Diffusion

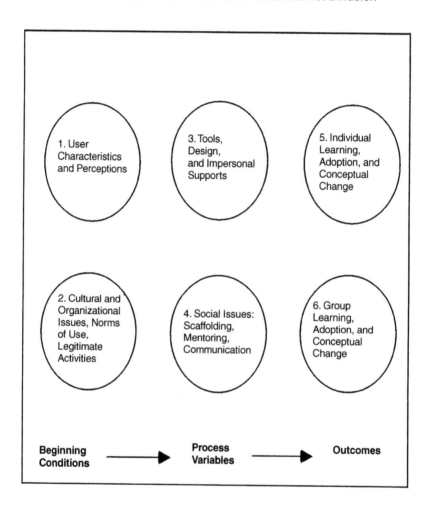

faculty and staff (Wilson, Ryder, McCahan, & Sherry, 1996), and two other members conducted focus groups with I.T. graduate students (Ryder & Wilson, 1996). Five factors emerged from these qualitative studies: (a) clear benefit and value, (b) self-efficacy, (c) finding a voice and having something to say (also referred to as mediated writing proficiency), (d) personal/cultural compatibility, and (e) proper scaffolding. Other researchers (Rogers, 1995; Bandura, 1982; Fishman, 1997; Berge, 1997; Hall & Hord, 1987) also identified these five factors.

TABLE 1. A Comparison of an Activity System and the Factors that Affect Internet Diffusion

Activity System	Clusters of Factors
Subject	User characteristics and perceptions, vision of learning
Rules	Cultural and organizational issues including norms and legitimate activities
Instruments	Tools, design, and impersonal supports
Division of labor	Social issues including roles, scaffolding, mentoring, and communication
Object or Outcome	Individual learning, adoption, and conceptual change
Community	Group learning, adoption, and conceptual change

In spring 1995, Sherry (1997) also conducted a survey of 73 members of the I.T. Division to ascertain their use of e-mail and the Internet for instructional purposes. Participants were asked about their role in the division (student, faculty, staff), access to technology that would support the use of Internet tools, patterns of use, reasons for use, facilitators and barriers, and rankings on eight proposed supports for training and performance using telecommunications. A factor analysis of the reasons for use, with Varimax rotation, resulted in four factors: share/disseminate information and communicate (41.5% of variance), find/organize information (11.7% of variance), collaborate (8.7% of variance), and consult with advisor (7.8% of variance). Responses to eleven challenges to use grouped into three factors: clear benefit and value (32.5% of variance), self-efficacy (17.2% of variance), and finding a voice and having something to say (10.4% of variance). These were three of the five factors that emerged from the focus groups with students and the interviews with faculty.

From the 1995 survey, the findings of the Internet Task Force, and the six clusters of factors influencing Internet diffusion that emerged from the literature review, ten research questions were created. These are presented in Table 2.

Current Design and Procedure

The current investigation began by triangulating the results from all of the published papers and internal documents produced between 1994 and 1997. In spring 1997, the 1995 survey was repeated using the same instrument (Sherry, 1998, Appendix C), but this time with a stratified

TABLE 2. Six Themes and Ten Research Questions

Theme	Research Questions
1. User characteristics and perceptions, vision of learning	1A. To what extent is the Internet used by the school?
	1B. For what reasons is the Internet used by the school?
	1C. What challenges to the use of the Internet are perceived as most important?
2. Cultural and organizational issues including norms and legitimate activities	2A. How does the incentive structure of the school influence the types and levels of use of the Internet?
	2B. What online activities are consonant with the administration's vision of disciplined inquiry, professional engagement, and professional leadership and commitment by faculty and graduate students?
3. Tools, design, and impersonal supports	3A. What improvements to the university network's human-computer interface design and available Internet tools are suggested by new and continuing users?
4. Social issues including roles, scaffolding, mentoring, and communication	4A. What changes to the school's communication and support structure are thought to be most helpful to overcome barriers and support Internet use?
	4B. How does the way that the school's members are joined to communication channels and other individuals influence their use of the Internet?
5. Individual learning, adoption, and conceptual change	5A. How do activities involving the use of Internet tools impact individual learning, adoption, and conceptual change?
6. Group learning, adoption, and conceptual change	6A. How does individual learning, adoption, and conceptual change influence the other members of the community to which these individuals are culturally linked?

random sample of 278 students, faculty, and staff taken from the nine divisions within the Graduate School of Education. The non-representative sample of the 1995 survey, which was limited to I.T. faculty, students, and staff, limited the generalizability of the initial findings. The stratified sample of the entire school in the 1997 survey was intended to alleviate this problem.

The 1997 survey sample consisted of about one-fifth males and four-fifths females, from entering masters students to tenured professors, and was representative of the School as a whole. The percentage of respondents from each division was approximately equal to the percentage of students enrolled in that division. I.T. respondents were separated from non-I.T. respondents. A factor analysis was performed on the new survey to investigate changes over time.

In spring 1998, a focus group was conducted with a cohort of non-I.T. students to offset the emphasis on the I.T. population. Twelve interviews were also conducted, recorded, transcribed, and analyzed, using a purposeful selection of students, faculty, and staff from several divisions within the school. Five early adopters, three early/late majority, and four resisters or "laggards" (Rogers, 1995) were interviewed. An investigation of electronic artifacts lent triangulation to this study and offset the emphasis on self-reported data. These artifacts consisted of archived e-mail messages from a spring 1997 class electronic conference, samples of student online portfolios, and samples of student and faculty Web pages. The data collection matrix is presented in Table 3.

Limitations of the Study

Construct validity is always a problem when dealing with affective measures. Here, it was strengthened by having the survey instrument evaluated and revised by a team of experts (the Internet Task Force), who were able to judge the extent to which the sample of items represented the defined domain. Reliability was strengthened by using a predefined protocol for guided interviews and the focus group. The instrument (Sherry, 1998, Appendix D) is highly structured and includes a large number of probes that are listed in the instrument itself.

RESULTS

Changes in Usage Over Time

In 1995, I.T. respondents primarily used the university UNIX system for their e-mail accounts, except for the few who had commercial or corporate accounts. By 1997, the variety of available tools had increased throughout the school; 86% of the respondents used e-mail; 74% used the WWW; and 60% used the electronic conferencing system.

Efficacy × Value

A factor analysis of the responses to the survey questions (Sherry, 1998, Appendix C) that dealt with reasons for using the Internet (14 items) and challenges to using the Internet (11 items) was performed for three subsets of data: (a) 1995 responses (all I.T.), (b) 1997 responses

TABLE 3. Data Collection Matrix

Question	1995 Survey	1997 Survey	Interviews	Focus Group	Electronic Artifacts
1A. To what extent is the Internet used by the SOE?	x	x	x	x	
1B. For what reasons is the Internet used by the SOE?	x	x	x	x	x
1C. What challenges to the use of the Internet are perceived as most important?	x	x	x	x	
2A. How does the incentive structure of the SOE influence the types and levels of use of the Internet?			x	x	
2B. What online activities are consonant with the administration's vision of disciplined inquiry, professional engagement, and professional leadership and commitment by faculty and graduate students?		x	x		x
3A. What improvements to the UCD and the SOE network's human-computer interface (HCI) design and available Internet tools are suggested by new and continuing users?	x	x	x	x	
4A. What changes to the UCD and the SOE's communication and support structure are thought to be most helpful to overcome barriers and support Internet use?	x	x	x	x	
4B. How does the way that SOE members are joined to communication channels and other individuals influence their use of the Internet?			x	x	x
5A. How do activities involving the use of Internet tools impact individual learning, adoption, and conceptual change?			x	x	x
6A. How does individual learning, adoption, and conceptual change influence the other members of the community to which these individuals are culturally linked?			x	x	x

(I.T.), and (c) 1997 responses (non-I.T.). A principal components analysis with Varimax rotation was then performed on the three sets of data. This revealed the general trends and changes over two years and also highlighted the differences between the I.T. and the non-I.T. sub-populations. The results are presented in Tables 4 and 5.

The primary reasons for Internet use: finding information, communicating with colleagues, sharing information, and collaboration (i.e., sharing information to carry out an intentional activity) varied in importance across time and between programs. In contrast, the facilitators to Internet use were remarkably consistent in all cases, with Bandura's efficacy $\times$ value accounting for about half the variance.

TABLE 4. Results of Factor Analysis on Reasons for Use

Survey	1995: I.T.	1997: I.T.	1997: Non-I.T.
Factor 1	Communicate and share information (42% of variance)	Share information (44% of variance)	Find information and collaborate (50% of variance)
Factor 2	Find information (12% of variance)	Communicate (11% of variance)	Share information (11% of variance)
Factor 3	Collaborate (9% of variance)	Collaborate (8% of variance)	Communicate (8% of variance)
Factor 4	Consult with advisor (8% of variance)	Find information (7% of variance)	

TABLE 5. Results of Factor Analysis on Facilitators to Use

Survey	1995: I.T.	1997: I.T.	1997: Non-I.T.
Factor 1	Clear benefit and value (33% of variance)	Clear benefit and value (32% of variance)	Clear benefit and value (38% of variance)
Factor 2	Self-efficacy (17% of variance)	Time and access (15% of variance)	Self-efficacy (16% of variance)
Factor 3	Mediated writing proficiency (10% of variance)	Self-efficacy part 1. (10.4% of variance)	
Factor 4		Self-efficacy part 2. (9% of variance)	

Personal/Cultural Compatibility

In the interviews, students, faculty, and staff alike reported that the e-mail feature of the electronic conferencing system was, and will continue to be, an efficient and convenient means of communication between students and faculty. Two faculty members also predicted that using distributed learning technologies might prove a viable alternative to traveling long distances in order to provide classes for geographically dispersed cohorts.

Responses from the focus group indicated that there was social pressure among some of the learning sub-communities within the school that reinforced the feeling of "If you don't participate, you may find yourself left behind." Both the interviews and the focus group presented evidence that the early adopters tended to be intrinsically motivated, whereas the later adopters often felt extrinsic coercion. Nearly all interviewees noted that there was no incentive system in place for them to adopt Internet tools other than e-mail. There was also some resistance to the idea of distance/distributed learning by both students and faculty.

Early adopters often expressed a good fit between Internet tools and their personal and cultural values. Late adopters voiced concerns about the impact of the Internet on teaching and learning. They felt that it may not support their vision of learning because it changes both the role of the instructor (Apple Computer, 1995; Yocam, 1998) and his/her core of instructional practice (Elmore, 1996).

Finding a Voice and Having Something to Say

From the perspectives of Diffusion Theory and Activity Theory, if Internet tools do not make communication easier for the user, then all the training in the world will not turn a resister into an adopter. Fishman (1997) found a significant negative relationship between written communication apprehension and the use of Usenet newsgroups among students who were using a combination of CMC tools in a mediated learning environment. Moreover, electronic communication is perceived by some learners to be more reflective than spoken interaction. "The very act of assembling one's thoughts and articulating them in writing for a [computer] conference audience appears to involve deeper cognitive processing" (Berge, 1997, p. 10). This is a factor that the Internet Task Force found in the 1995 interviews. It also showed up as the Factor 3 in the 1995 survey factor analysis.

By 1997, this factor had disappeared from the survey results, but it was still reported by two interviewees. A student alluded to new forms of literacy that needed to be explored and developed: visual literacy, media literacy, and literacy in terms of the Internet and e-mail. A faculty member discussed the additional cognitive skills that are necessary when dealing with online documents. Some faculty members did use electronic conferencing, but not all were aware of the possibilities that this new form of interactive communication and instruction might entail.

Electronic artifacts, other than archived messages from class electronic conferences, were sparse. Out of the entire Graduate School of Education, few members contributed to the school's online scholarly publications (9 faculty, 20 students), and fewer used personal Web pages to disseminate full-text versions of their publications (3 faculty, 8 students). One explanatory factor might be fear among students and faculty of compromising intellectual property rights; but concerns about ownership and copyright issues did not surface in any of the interviews.

Proper Scaffolding and Support

Existing and proposed supports were divided into two categories: impersonal and personal. Impersonal supports comprised brochures, booklets, online tutorials, and other forms of print-based or electronic performance support that do not require one-on-one interaction with a graduate assistant, fellow student, faculty member, or staff member. Personal supports comprised help from graduate assistants, online help from the university's Computing, Information, and Network Services (CINS) staff, direct instruction in class, and free workshops conducted by faculty, staff, technically adept students, or other perceived experts.

Interview participants were asked to suggest improvements to the school's support structure. Survey participants were asked to rank a set of eight supports for training and performance. In both the 1995 and 1997 surveys, the results were confounded in a few cases by about 5% of the participants who rated, rather than ranked, the suggested supports.

In 1995, formal classes and workshops were ranked highest; booklets were ranked lowest; and individual attention by graduate students was bipolar. There were significant but low positive Spearman correlations ($p < .05$) between the self-efficacy factor and the relative rankings of both formal classes ($r = .026$) and individual attention by graduate students ($r = .029$). There was a significant but low negative correlation ($p < .05$) between the self-efficacy factor and the relative ranking of informative booklets ($r = -.025$). This led to the conclusion that respondents who were low in self-efficacy considered personal supports and scaffolding to be relatively useful as compared with impersonal supports such as booklets.

In 1997, formal classes and workshops were still ranked highest; booklets were still ranked lowest; and the bipolarity in the ranking for individual attention by graduate assistants disappeared. In contrast, online tutorials were now bipolar. These rankings indicated that the respondents generally preferred personal scaffolding to impersonal supports, but held varying opinions concerning the specific type of support that they would like to see implemented.

Faculty and students alike were often unaware of the range of supports that existed. For example, the university's computing staff had already developed an extensive set of free workshops–exactly the type of 1- or 2-hour workshops that students requested. Brochures, schedules, and job aids explaining various facets of the university's computers and directions for using them were freely available at the university's computer center and at the Graduate School of Education's computer laboratory. However, the students and staff were apparently not aware of these instructional materials, and graduate assistants did not publicize them to new users. An important aspect of an activity system is the fact that for it to function efficiently, information must flow freely throughout the system, to and from all participants. If a support exists, but users are not aware of it, then it is like not being there at all!

RECOMMENDATIONS

Based on the results of this study, recommendations for future investigation and development are listed in Table 6. Some of these recommendations were collected from responses to the final question on the survey, "What other suggestions do you have for us?" The majority of the recommendations were taken from the transcripts of the interviews with students, faculty, and staff. Other colleges and universities that are considering using the Internet and the WWW to enhance instruction might find them applicable as well.

IMPLICATIONS

Based on this study's findings, the use of e-mail will continue to increase because the electronic conferencing system has become com-

TABLE 6. Recommendations

Have better publicity about existing aids and supports, using multiple channels of communication.

Have better communication and collaboration between the Graduate School of Education, the university, and the university's Computing, Information, and Network Services (CINS), possibly sharing duties where they overlap.

Develop a flexible schedule of electronic conferencing demonstrations or open lab workshops with optional student attendance.

Hire more graduate students in the Graduate School of Education computer lab who have the skills and the time to help individual students with specific problems.

Create a permanent position for an in-building technical support person who will be available in person or by telephone when classes are in session.

Encourage "show and tell" sessions among faculty members to discuss and share ideas, strategies, and promising practices for Internet use beyond simple e-mail messaging to support teaching and learning.

Encourage students to create online research management products and portfolios to serve as models of scholarly products for new students, and to elicit feedback from peers, colleagues, and experts.

monly accepted throughout the school. All interviewees and focus group members used the conferencing system regularly in 1997, in contrast with the more sporadic e-mail use in 1995. Students in the focus group stated that it was more convenient to connect from home or work on a regular basis rather than to travel to campus and pay for parking.

Use of the WWW continues to increase, since Internet service is now provided for all registered students through their fees. Students who primarily used the electronic conferencing system discovered that it did not automatically provide the same types of Internet-wide search engines and database tools as the WWW. They stated that they would like better access to research-based databases, online libraries, collections of legal and medical information, and other resources that are freely available on the WWW, which matched their own educational goals. Additionally, many new students are already Internet enculturated. According to one of the interviewed staff, one out of four applicants in spring 1998 were from out of state and found out about the school's programs via the Web page that was created by the Internet Task Force.

As a result of this study, both the Graduate School of Education and the university have become more aware that no electronic help-desk can offer the type of support that new users need as they deal with their personal and task management concerns (Hall & Hord, 1997). Some of the recommendations presented here have already been incorporated. For example, the Teaching and Learning with Technology (TLT) laboratory was recently created for the purpose of mentoring faculty in the use of telecommunications and educational technology. The university's Office of Teaching Effectiveness offers a summer Boot Camp for Professors. This week-long conference stresses the use of new technologies to enhance teaching and learning, and has gained popularity in recent years. Based on student and faculty requests for one-on-one scaffolding, the Office of Teaching Effectiveness created a new work-study program in June 1999. A cohort of incoming freshmen was trained as the "Student Instructional Technology Corps." This training enabled them to serve as technical assistants to various academic divisions throughout the university.

Increased usage will not come without unintended side effects. What is working now may not work in the future. Students with slow modems and insufficient RAM are beginning to feel a sense of frustration with their older hardware platforms. Students in rural areas or new suburban subdivisions do not have access to DSL (a high-speed digital communications service). As new users come on board, especially those who are unfamiliar with computer-mediated communication, they continue to have problems with modem settings and other software issues.

System overload, too, may present a problem as more and more students begin to use their free student accounts to access the WWW. The university's server capacity will be stressed, leading to an increase in carrier drops and busy signals. All of this can be frustrating for new and experienced users alike. The university, like other educational organizations (Sherry, Lawyer-Brook, & Black, 1997), has had to increase its server capacity and purchase additional servers to keep up with increased online traffic as new users connect on a regular basis. Any program or educational institution will eventually have to deal with these issues as they progress through the stages of adoption, implementation, and institutionalization of Internet tools that support and deliver instruction.

REFERENCES

Apple Computer. (1995). *Changing the conversation about teaching, learning, and technology: A report on 10 years of ACOT research* [Online]. Available: *http://www.research.apple.com/go/acot/ACOTResearch.html*

Bandura, A. (1982). Self-efficacy mechanism in human agency. *American Psychologist, 37* (2), 122-147.

Berge, Z. (1997). Computer conferencing and the on-line classroom. *International Journal of Educational Telecommunications, 3*(1), 3-21.

Elmore, R.F. (1996). Getting to scale with good educational practice. *Harvard Educational Review, 66*(1), 1-26.

Engestrom, Y. (1996). Interobjectivity, ideality, and dialectics. *Mind, Culture, and Activity, 3*(4), 259-265.

Engestrom, Y. (1998). *Activity Theory.* [Online]. Available: *http://www.helsinki. fi/~jengestr/activity/6b.htm*

Fishman, B.J. (1997, March). *Student traits and the use of computer-mediated communication tools: What matters and why?* Paper presented at the Annual Meeting of the American Educational Research Association, Chicago, IL.

Hall, G.E., & Hord, S.M. (1987). *Change in schools: Facilitating the process.* Albany, NY: State University of New York Press.

Rogers, E.M. (1995). *Diffusion of innovations (4th Edition).* New York: The Free Press.

Ryder, M., & Wilson, B. (1996, February). *Affordances and constraints of the Internet for learning and instruction.* Paper presented at the annual meeting of the Association for Educational Communications and Technology, Indianapolis, IN.

Sherry, L. (1998). *Diffusion of the Internet within a graduate school of education* (Doctoral dissertation, University of Colorado at Denver, 1998). UMI, 300 North Zeeb Road, Ann Arbor MI 48106-1346. [Online]. Available: *http://www.cudenver. edu/~lsherry/dissertation/*

Sherry, L. (1997). *A re-analysis of the 1995 TSS e-mail survey* [Online]. Available: *http://www.cudenver.edu/public/education/sherry/95survey.html*

Sherry, L., Lawyer-Brook, D., & Black, L. (1997). Evaluation of the Boulder Valley Internet Project: A theory-based approach to evaluation design. *Journal of Interactive Learning Research, 8*(2), 199-233.

Sherry, L., & Myers, K.M. (1998). The dynamics of collaborative design. *IEEE Transactions on Professional Communication, 41*(2), 123-139.

Sherry, L., & the UCD Internet Task Force. (1996). Supporting a networked community of learners. *TechTrends, 1*(4), 28-32.

Tikhomirov, O.K. (1981). The psychological consequences of computerization. In J.V. Wertsch (Ed.), *The concept of activity in Soviet psychology* (pp. 256-278). Armonk, NY: M.E. Sharpe.

Wilson, B., Lowry, M., Koneman, P., & Osman-Jouchoux, R. (1994). *Electronic discussion groups: Using e-mail as an instructional strategy in a graduate seminar* [Online]. Available: *http://www.cudenver.edu/public/education/edschool/email.html*

Wilson, B., Ryder, M., McCahan, J., & Sherry, L. (1996). Cultural assimilation of the Internet: A case study. In M. Simonson (Ed.), *Proceedings of selected research and development presentations.* Washington, DC: Association for Educational Communications and Technology.

Yocam, K. (1998). *Teacher-centered staff development* [Online document]. Available: *http://www.apple.com/education/k12/staffdev/tchrcenterstaff.html*

Eric Reynolds
Diana Treahy
Chin-chi Chao
Sasha Barab

The Internet Learning Forum: Developing a Community Prototype for Teachers of the 21st Century

SUMMARY. This paper reports an effort to create a community of practice for teachers' professional development via the World Wide Web. Beginning with a discussion of our theoretical foundations and current online models of professional development, we address the problem of how developing Web and video technologies may provide innovative and effective professional development for teachers. We describe the initial conceptions of the Internet Learning Forum (ILF), a Web site

ERIC REYNOLDS is MS, Language Education Department, Wright Building, Room 3044, 201 North Rose Avenue, Indiana University, Bloomington, IN 47405 (E-mail: edreynol@alumni.indiana.edu).
DIANA TREAHY is Doctoral Student, Mathematics Education, Department of Curriculum and Instruction, Wright Building, Room 3056, 201 North Rose Avenue, Indiana University, Bloomington, IN 47405 (E-mail: dtreahy@indiana.edu).
CHIN-CHI CHAO is Doctoral Candidate, Language Education Department, Wright Building, Room 3044, 201 North Rose Avenue, Indiana University, Bloomington, IN 47405 (E-mail: cchao@indiana.edu).
SASHA BARAB is Assistant Professor, Department of Instructional Systems Technology, Wright Building, Room 2232, 201 North Rose Avenue, Indiana University, Bloomington, IN 47405 (E-mail: sbarab@indiana.edu).

[Haworth co-indexing entry note]: "The Internet Learning Forum: Developing a Community Prototype for Teachers of the 21st Century." Reynolds, Eric et al. Co-published simultaneously in *Computers in the Schools* (The Haworth Press, Inc.) Vol. 17, No. 3/4, 2001, pp. 107-125; and: *The Web in Higher Education: Assessing the Impact and Fulfilling the Potential* (ed: Cleborne D. Maddux, and D. LaMont Johnson) The Haworth Press, Inc., 2001, pp. 107-125. Single or multiple copies of this article are available for a fee from The Haworth Document Delivery Service [1-800-342-9678, 9:00 a.m. - 5:00 p.m. (EST). E-mail address: getinfo@haworthpressinc.com].

107

developed to support mathematics and science teachers sharing and evolving their pedagogical practices. This site includes exemplary instructional units, teachers' reflections, and peer discussion. Starting with video, ILF participants examine assumptions, reflect on practices, and share within the ILF community. The goal of this unique community of practice is to create quality professional development. While this paper provides an overview of our initial design work, the site has evolved into a nationally funded project. However, the work described here, which guided the development of the prototype, has important implications for other Web-based efforts to support teacher professional development. *[Article copies available for a fee from The Haworth Document Delivery Service: 1-800-342-9678. E-mail address: <getinfo@haworthpressinc.com> Website: <http://www.HaworthPress.com> © 2001 by The Haworth Press, Inc. All rights reserved.]*

KEYWORDS. Community of practice, online community, professional development, Internet, multimedia, reflective teaching, teacher education, instructional systems, educational innovation

The difficulty of implementing change in education has been widely discussed in recent years. Traditionally, approaches to teacher development have assumed a stance toward teaching practice that concentrated on answers: conveying information, providing ideas, training in skills (Ball, 1996; Willis, 1997). In addition, Chism (1985) indicates that, while the notions of peer interaction and support within the school and community of teachers are well understood, and indeed most teachers claim to practice them, ethnographic observation has found a significant lack of professional peer interaction among teachers in public schools (Darling-Hammond, 1996). Consequently, a lack of critical reflective discussion among teachers has existed, and generally teachers find themselves developing their practice in isolation or at in-service workshops. Additionally, support for change is rarely ongoing and rarely situated in the immediate pedagogical needs of the teachers (Smylie & Conyers, 1991).

Barab and Duffy (2000) point out that traditional approaches to teacher development often fail because they do not create a sense of community that values and engages in reflection on the teacher's own classroom practice. Furthermore, the lack of pedagogical models for teacher professional development that move from a didactic approach to a learning-as-part-of-a-community approach hampers reform efforts.

Most critically, change has been slow simply because the culture of sharing pedagogical strategies is not well-established. Clearly, new models for professional development are needed, models that foster a culture of sharing and provide sustained communal support for teachers as they evaluate both their beliefs and practices.

The project we describe here is the creation of a virtual community on the World Wide Web designed to support the professional development of teachers. We call the community the Internet Learning Forum, or ILF. The project is based on the design efforts of the 24 members of the ILF prototype team. The design of this virtual community was guided by theoretical research on situated learning, and community building structures, as well as current virtual models for professional development. Practical concerns drawn from analyzing the teaching contexts of community members also shaped the project: specifically, available technology, professional standards, licensure requirements, and the teacher's own needs. Exploring these elements resulted in four fundamental principles for the ILF. Ultimately, the project itself is our attempt to integrate these elements.

THEORETICAL BACKGROUND

The theoretical underpinnings of this project grow out of situated cognition theory, into communities of practice, and, finally, into an exploration of Web-based professional development models. Much of situated cognition theory is based on observing learning in everyday activities and apprenticeships, and on the wealth of research that has found that content learned in the context of schools frequently fails to transfer when students enter out-of-school contexts (Brown, Collins, & Duguid, 1989; Greeno, 1998; Lave, 1993). Researchers emphasize engaging in real-world practices, partly for the reason that students can get the intact, spontaneous, sometimes hidden, wisdom from experts and practitioners, just as apprentices do with their mentors. Brown and Duguid (1989) also maintain that everyday activities situated in the cultures in which people work allow students to develop matured proficiency through observing how experts engage in intuitive reasoning, problem solving, and meaning negotiating.

Real-world problems arise in a particular context and are resolved within the constraints of those contexts. Becoming knowledgeably skillful necessitates not simply developing specific skills but having a contextualized appreciation for how those skills relate to actual practice. Thus, being deprived of the opportunity of interacting with real professionals in an authentic context and activity, students are likely to engage in what Brown et al. called "ersatz activities" and, consequently, develop incomplete conceptions of the practice and the domain. Opportunities for pre-service and in-service teachers to situate their learning in real-world practices and classrooms are important (Barab, Squire, & Dueber, 2000).

A concept that can guide the design of teacher professional development programs, according to some situated cognition theorists, is community of practice (Barab, Cherkes-Julkowski, Swenson, Garrett, Shaw, & Young, 1999; Barab & Duffy, 2000). Barab and Duffy (2000) described a community as having three components. First, a community has a significant history and a shared cosmology, especially related to shared goals, practices, belief systems, and collective stories that capture canonical practices. Second, the notion of community suggests something larger than any one member. Third, a community is constantly reproducing itself such that new members contribute, support, and eventually lead the community into the future. In a community of practice, novices have the opportunity to participate in real-world practices alongside experts and professionals as, what Lave and Wenger call, "legitimate peripheral participants" (Lave & Wenger, 1991). Indeed, research in professional development indicates that the most effective professional development occurs when formal instruction is supported by informal community structures (Lagache, 1993; Seely-Brown, 1998). To engage in community of practice is important for both pre-service and in-service teachers' professional development throughout their careers.

Our belief is that technological innovations on the Internet create new opportunities for supporting the development of a community of practice and for situating teacher professional development in classroom contexts. Particularly, we see the potential of allowing teachers from different contexts to form a community of practice, which can greatly benefit teachers in their professional development. As far as we can observe, the Web has enabled at least four different models of teacher professional development: a skill-based training model, student inquiry projects model, spontaneous participation model, and distance education course model. In the next section we briefly review these models.

FOUR ONLINE MODELS
OF PROFESSIONAL DEVELOPMENT

Skill-Based Training Model

Skill-based training presents a specific set of knowledge, skills, or information in more or less sequenced lessons, often patterned as a workshop or a collection of resources. The learning is self-paced, and answers are provided to specific questions that teachers might have. Some examples follow:

1. Link2learn–Workshop Kits
   http://l2lpd.arin.k12.pa.us/workkits/
2. How to Make a Successful ESL/EFL Teacher's Web Page, by Charles Kelly
   http://www.aitech.ac.jp/~iteslj/Articles/Kelly-MakePage/
3. Science and Math Initiative: Math, Science, and Classroom Resources
   http://www.learner.org/sami/

The training model does not usually include the opportunity for collaboration or interaction among teachers or the opportunity for reflection on practices. The model is focused on transferring skills and information. The danger is that it can limit the teacher's view to narrow content. For example, many Web training programs on computer skills tend to focus on nothing but technology and its functions, rather than encouraging teachers to consider how to properly incorporate technology based on their curricular needs. Successful use of this kind of skill-based model requires that learners consciously fill in the gaps and make the information useful in their respective context.

Student Inquiry Projects Model

Popularity of the Internet has encouraged inquiry project collaboration among students from different regions or parts of the world. For example, Ruopp and his colleagues in TERC, Inc., organized a series of scientific projects that puts students in the position of scientists working with scientists (Ruopp, Gal, Drayton, & Pfister, 1993). Many of these projects require that the teachers of participating classes work closely together in making project decisions, solving problems, and negotiating for the details of the project. That participating teachers exchange insight and information is therefore a natural part of the project–a part that gradually becomes strong support for professional development. The student project thus is an opportunity for teachers to grow profession-ally by actually negotiating and engaging with other teachers. They de-pend on help from colleagues to develop expertise in guiding the students and managing the project, to reflect on their own practices, to examine their assumptions, and to develop their own technological pro-ficiency. The rich learning, interaction, and reflection opportunities are congruent with many professional development standards for teachers.

The student project model is ideal for in-service teachers but may not work for pre-service teachers, because it requires that the teacher has his or her own student group, which most pre-service teachers do not have. According to the community of practice concept, providing members the opportunity to participate is essential, but how best to accomplish that participation is the subject of this project.

Spontaneous Participation Model

A third kind of Internet professional development opportunity allows teachers to participate whenever they have some free time. An example is TAPPEDIN (*http://www.tappedin.sri.com/*), which is an Internet vir-tual environment that takes the metaphor of a conference center. Orga-nizations such as the National Science Foundation, Geological Society of America, and many others hold online offices, meetings, and projects there for users to engage in real-time (synchronous) collaboration. Gatherings of general purposes are also provided to all the teacher members in the community, such as the After-School Online Discus-sions. Users can send e-mail, post to bulletin boards and listservs (asynchronously), and browse Web sites together as a group. They also have the choice of following the discussion closely or participating only when they feel the need.

Although many opportunities exist for individuals to participate and exchange information, a potential weakness of this model is that, when commitment is lacking, the learning may be loose and does not last long. Also, a short online meeting often does not allow participants to fully discuss an issue. Another problem is that participants may not ac-cess the site at the right time for the needed discussion. To benefit from the experience, it may require strong motivation, interest, commitment, and consistent participation, which are quite different from the intention of keeping the opportunity flexible enough for people to participate spontaneously. TAPPEDIN tries to solve this problem by providing regular e-mail notices which, however, are not always effective in encouraging commitment and participation. Commitment may be enhanced when the user can rely on the quality of information offered by the site. Many teachers rely on such content-focused sites as the Math Forum (*http://forum.swarthmore.edu/*) for that precise reason.

Distance Education Course Model

Another recent popular choice for teacher professional development is the Web-based distance education course. These courses use the Internet as the medium for instruction and interaction, using a combination of technologies such as printed text, hypertext, Web scripting, audio, video, e-mail, and synchronous and asynchronous conferencing tools. An example is a series of distance education courses offered by the School of Education at Indiana University (*http://www.indiana. edu/~disted/*). Teachers do not need to leave their jobs to get accredited courses that are required for certification or license renewal. They can attend the class any time that is convenient to them, and the course requirements and structure can often create a commitment. The distance nature of the course can also bring together participants with much more varied backgrounds than conventional classroom courses. Interaction with colleagues from diverse backgrounds is possible to help expand the participants' perspectives in many different ways.

Given the large number of courses being offered by different universities, colleges, and private organizations from all over the world, confirming quality is so far a challenge for users. For example, some courses are similar to traditional correspondence courses that do not allow the important opportunities of interaction and reflection with colleagues. Consumers must be alert in selecting courses. As discussed above, each of these models has its strengths and weaknesses. Our goal, then, has been to create learning opportunities that combine the advantages of all of the described models–and eliminate as many disadvantages as possible–and to seek to fill in gaps in meeting professional standards.

FUNDAMENTAL PRINCIPLES

In creating the Internet-based professional development tool, we have incorporated elements of the four models–skill-based training, student inquiry projects, spontaneous participation, and distance education courses–into the ILF. The in-depth resources central to a skills-based environment have been placed in the ILF resource room. The rich learning, interaction, and reflection opportunities central to the inquiry model are developed in the professional interaction found in the discussions of individual lessons and on specific topics of interest. The flexible and spontaneous participation found in such high-quality, high-reputation, spontaneous participation model sites such as the Math Forum, is found in asynchronous discussions with professors and peers. The flexible, yet structured, benefits of distance education coursework are found in teacher training courses currently being designed for the ILF. By synthesizing the best elements of all four models, we seek to build on these already successful projects. In designing this environment, we drew on this synthesis and the below discussed three design principles: visit the classroom, grow the community, and foster ownership and participation. Last, there were several practical concerns and opportunities that informed our design work.

Visit the Classroom

The goal of situating the participants in the social context of the practice was central to the design of the ILF. Observation and reflection are powerful modes of learning. Further, the craft of teaching consists, in large part, of tacit skills and knowledge that are not easily shared in words alone. Hence, an important starting point for sharing practices in a community of teacher practitioners is through visiting one another's classrooms to observe the craft of teaching as a basis for analysis, discussion, and reflection. To achieve this metaphorical classroom visit, supporting members of the community share videos of their own teaching practices.

While video has been used for decades in teacher training, the potential of this medium has not been optimized in online professional development settings. Reynolds and O'Neil (1997) noted how video technology remedies several difficulties associated with in-service teacher development. They observed that even teaching at the same school, teachers found it difficult to find time to observe other teachers' classes. Video allows for the capturing of instruction until both the teacher and the observers find time to sit down and explore the practice. Reynolds and O'Neil (1997) emphasized that working together to analyze instruction using the videotape fostered community building among teachers. They reported that social interaction between teachers increased and that a greater sense of community within the institution was found.

The strategy for employing videos is based on the design of the multimedia system, Strategic Teaching Framework (STF) (Duffy, 1997). The STF employs the "visit-the-classroom" metaphor, where a teacher virtually sits in on a class, pausing at any time to get different perspectives on class activities. She may also link her comments to the video and, when issues arise, access a rich database on teaching strategies. Chaney (1995) described elementary school teachers collaboratively using STF to analyze and critique exemplary instruction demonstrated by model teachers captured on videodisc. Observing teachers watched the demonstration and then had the chance to hear the demonstrating teachers' reflections on the viewed segment afterwards. The video captured the model teachers' moment-to-moment decision-making process, while the discussion among observing teachers after viewing the video clip helped them critically review their own assumptions about teaching and learning and improve their practices. Evaluation of the STF has demonstrated its effectiveness in both pre-service instruction (Lambdin, Duffy, & Moore, 1997) and in-service support for change (Chaney-Cullen & Duffy, 1998).

A critical issue in this project was understanding what representations and participant structures support the sharing of (making explicit) tacit knowledge (Brown & Duguid, 1998). Videos provide a start, but context and an interpretive frame are certainly needed. Thus, the videos are seen as a jumping-off point for discussions about the practice, including discussion of video use in different contexts, its relation to other practices, artifacts from the episode, and, eventually, discussion of attempts to implement or adopt the practice.

Grow the Community

It is *not* our notion that we will "build it, and they will come." Instead, initially we intend to create links with already existing communities, meeting their existing needs and building on their existing relations. For example, one way to create a culture of ongoing professional sharing and collaboration is to establish such professional sharing and collaboration as an expectation from the beginning of pre-service teacher education. The culture of sharing and discussing teaching practices, and the ILF as a tool to support that activity, will be introduced during undergraduate teacher education. Thus, our hope is that the community established on campus will rapidly grow into off-campus, in-service communities. Further, the size of the community, even focusing on only math and science teaching, offers a rich research environment in assessing the social, psychological, and technological issues in establishing and sustaining communities.

A critical issue in growing the community also involves supporting the transition process and responding to the changing needs of individuals as they move from the university campus to the K-12 school environment. While we will have established the culture of sharing, the relevant issues for discussion and sharing will change as individuals move into the teaching environment. Further, the world of work will offer less time for community participation. We examined two related strategies for sustaining participation during this transition and beyond. First, the design is based on enlisting core members of the mathematics and science teaching professional associations in the state to become active participants in the ILF–serving as "old timers" in the profession. Additionally, we discussed establishing face-to-face meetings among ILF community members in association with the professional meetings.

Foster Ownership and Participation

We believe that a truly effective and sustained professional development environment must be distributed throughout a community of professional practitioners of varied and wide experience and skill, who accept responsibility for building and maintaining the environment. In other words, the model must encourage a high degree of ownership and commitment, thereby bringing about participation. Professional development is not something that others "do" to teachers; rather, it is part and parcel of their individual and collective professional identity. Contributions to the system (e.g., new video episodes, revisions to system design, rules for participation) arise from the participants–a unique partnership of in-service teachers, pre-service teachers, teacher educators, researchers, technologists, etc.

A second factor that we think will drive teacher ownership and participation is the previously mentioned change in Indiana teacher licensure policy. We are confident that the requirement to include a teaching video in each teacher's licensure portfolio will reinforce the desire to participate in a community and contribute examples of teaching practices for discussion. Finally, the intent of the new professional teaching standards to actively evaluate teaching practices, along with the discipline-based standards, will serve as a major factor in determining the practices teachers will want to see and share. From a research perspective, we evaluate the degree to which establishing the culture of sharing in the pre-service and early years of teaching and the linkages to professional associations will provide the foundation for sustaining continued participation in the community.

PRACTICAL CONSTRAINTS AND OPPORTUNITIES

One practical concern is incorporating and integrating the professional standards and guidelines that define much of the American teaching practice. In 1994, Indiana adopted the Interstate New Teacher Assessment and Support Consortium (INTASC) performance-based standards model (1991). INTASC is a program to enhance collaboration among states interested in rethinking teacher assessment for initial licensing as well as for preparation and induction into the education profession. Several of these standards impinge directly on the ILF. Standard nine of the Professional Standards for the Mathematics Specialist Credential states, "teachers of mathematics are reflective practitioners who continually evaluate the effects of their choices and actions on others . . . and who actively seek out opportunities to grow professionally" (Indiana Professional Standards Board, 1996, p. 12). Thus, every teacher working under INTASC is mandated to seek out opportunities for reflective professional growth. Further, teachers are asked to "model improved practices" and "draw upon . . . learned societies as supports for reflection, problem solving, new ideas, sharing experiences, and participating in workshops and courses related to mathematics" (1996, p. 12). Clearly, INTASC urges full participation in the wider community of teaching practice.

Another factor influencing design of the prototype is the change in Indiana teacher licensure policy. Under the new policy, graduates are given an interim teaching license. During the two years after graduation, teachers must develop a portfolio demonstrating their competency, with a permanent license awarded based on the quality of that portfolio. A video of teaching is a key element of that portfolio requirement. This new requirement creates a need to participate in a community and contribute examples of teaching practices. The current demands for professional growth and standard-based credentialing requirements in Indiana and nationwide create pressing needs to evaluate the present situation in professional development programs and examine whether the existing programs are able to meet these needs.

The final practical concern was the teacher's self-defined needs. To determine what teachers want in an online professional development community, we surveyed and interviewed pre-service, novice and experienced teachers. Each group answered the same questions, using a combination of written surveys and one-on-one interviews. As a whole, the respondents spoke of needing to network with their peers and with more experienced teachers, and to some extent university faculty. The pre-service teachers interviewed and surveyed expressed a strong interest to work more extensively with senior teachers. Novice teachers found that working with their peers and with their "mentor" teachers (senior teachers assigned to work closely with first-year teachers in this state), proved the most important channel for professional development. Experienced teachers also rated working with peers as a vital part of their professional development, but in the case of these senior teachers, networking at professional conferences and workshops superseded in importance networking at the school site.

Similarly, the teachers surveyed wanted teacher resources to be provided by a professional development tool. Again, the nature of those resources differed between the experience groups. As mentioned previously, resources for workshops and conferences were most important for senior teachers. Novice and pre-service teachers looked for resources to meet their daily needs, such as lesson plans, unit plans, and background research on specific topics. A minority of respondents stated the need for special resources that might be difficult for a school site to provide, such as assistance with resources for special education students, links to teachers organizations, and assistance with legal issues.

A final theme consistent across all experience levels was that of connecting the professional development activities to "real" classroom experience. Experienced teachers talked of ensuring the transfer of new ideas to real classrooms. Novice teachers needed a virtual, human guide, and live interaction with teachers via chat or e-mail. Pre-service teachers wanted discussions with other teachers and direct feedback on classroom issues and experiences. Thus, incorporating community, resources, and direct connections to actual classroom experiences, became a priority for the design project.

THE INTERNET LEARNING FORUM

With an understanding of the theoretical research and the practical concerns drawn from analyzing the teaching contexts, as well as the fundamental principles for the ILF, a description of the preliminary product of the ILF prototype is in order. To design the site, three task groups were formed: content, video, and interface. The content team focused on issues of inclusion for such items as lesson and unit plans, professional and subject area standards, teacher and student reflections, and which clips of lessons to highlight. The video team dealt with aspects regarding the legal issues and permission forms required for videotaping children and publishing these clips on the Internet. This team was also responsible for all of the technical aspects behind capturing video in the classroom, digitizing the videotape, and then making it available on the Web through the use of video-streaming technology. The interface development team was responsible for developing the design and navigation of the site.

The heart of the site is the video of classroom instruction, which is designed to stimulate discussion related to teaching and learning among teacher participants. As an initial effort, we presented video segments of four practicing teachers as they gave unscripted math or science instruction in the classroom. Content team members worked with these teachers to choose the particular video segments from their lessons and presented these with the teacher's written comments, reflection, lesson plan, and matching professional standards in the Web site.

A brief description of the site is in order. The navigation of the site is relatively simple. The home page shows a virtual school with doors to a variety of offices (see Figure 1).

For the prototype, only math and science subject areas were included. Other administrative help can be found in the office and resource rooms. Teachers can meet and share their views in the teacher's lounge where Web-based conferencing tools are provided. Entering through either the math or science doors allows teacher participants to search for lessons by the demonstrating teacher's name, the instructional topic, or grade level (see Figure 2).

They can also browse through the video library. After selecting a classroom and lesson, participants will be taken directly to a classroom page (see Figure 3).

On that page participants can access the video as well as all of the text data for the lesson, including comments and reflections by the demonstrating teacher. As the information presented is about real classroom interactions with the demonstrating teachers working with their children, a password is required for participants to access the video image. Discussions and sharing occur on that page in relation to each video clip.

How will ILF users respond to the three fundamental community-building elements (visiting a classroom, building community, and fostering ownership and participation)? Ultimately, that is a question for

FIGURE 1. ILF Home Page

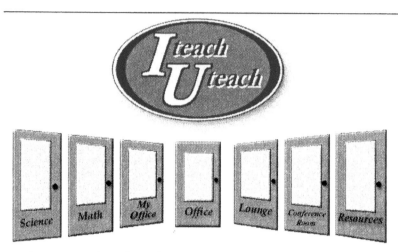

A community of teachers working and learning together ...

Visitors please check in at the main office. Thanks!

This page last updated
Internet Learning Forum @ Indiana University
Contact the ILF Development Team at ilf@indiana.edu

future research, but we should explore how they respond to our efforts to actualize those notions. Clearly, they will recognize the "visit-the-classroom" metaphor that situates this project in practical teaching experience and actual classrooms as an element that makes it real for the teacher participants. While our motivation as teacher educators is to provide teachers with professional development opportunities, the teachers also expressed a variety of real-world needs for their classroom teaching. Lesson plans, conference and workshop information, as well as special needs are provided for in the lesson areas, the teacher's lounge area, and the office area, respectively, of the ILF. Additionally, we are aware that teachers are more likely to choose a single site to meet their teaching needs if the information provided is rich and comprehensive. For this reason, our teacher's lounge is designed to include links to other sites that provide direct links to other subject area sites, as well as to sites of research institutions and foundations. Key to this learning environment is how the continual update process of site development, combined with

FIGURE 2. Classroom Selection Page

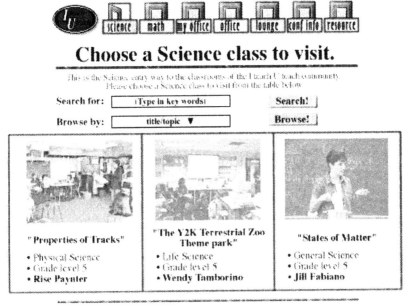

Choose a Science class to visit.

This is the Science entry way to the classrooms of the Teach Teach community. Please choose a Science class to visit from the table below.

Search for: [Type in key words]   Search!

Browse by: [title/topic ▼]   Browse!

"Properties of Tracks"	"The Y2K Terrestrial Zoo Theme park"	"States of Matter"
• Physical Science	• Life Science	• General Science
• Grade level 5	• Grade level 5	• Grade level 5
• Rise Paynter	• Wendy Tamborino	• Jill Fabiano

© Internet Learning Forum; Indiana University
Contact the ILF Development Team at crlt@indiana.edu

the immediacy of revision on the site, allows us maintain the site in ways that print documents could never accomplish. Moreover, the participants will be encouraged to add new information, share new lessons within the community, and ultimately create the most current environment for teacher resources and professional development.

The next issue of growing the community implies that we are supporting member participation and not information dissemination. Central to the design of the ILF is to establish participant structures, not "black boxed" resources. It is our belief that one cannot mandate community; instead, we view that our job is to design responsive structures that facilitate participation and are easily modifiable based on the needs of the participants. However, if we are going to encourage participation, we must provide a structure that is compelling enough to draw in participants.

FIGURE 3. Virtual Classroom Page

Clip 1: "What is a variable?"
(click to view)

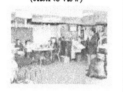

Choose a segment:

"What is a variable?"
"Evidence"
"What if we release the ball?"
"Student Questions"
"Discussion"

More Info:

Teacher Reflection
Overview of Lesson
Lesson/Unit Plan
Resources
Integration Ideas
Professional Standards
Discussion

science | math | my office | office | lounge | conf info | resource

Lesson Plan: Properties of Tracks

This is the 2nd lesson in this unit.

Materials: Small and large spheres, carbon paper, white paper, and a ramp, science logs, pencil

What are some questions you might try to find answers to using these materials?
1.
2.
3.
4.
When you do experiments you have constants and one variable? Can you think of one variable?
If the sphere size is different, everything else needs to stay the same. If the ramp release height is different then you would need the sphere size to stay the same. Ramp height changes, two large spheres.

Today we'll do one experiment -- everyone will test one variable -- the sphere size. (Handout sheets)

© Internet Learning Forum, Indiana University
Contact the ILF Development Team at crlt@indiana.edu

The ILF's Web-based conferencing functions have the ability to connect, for example, a teacher in a rural school–who may be the only teacher in their grade level or subject area at the school–to other teachers across the state. Additionally, the ILF classroom videos will provide newer and standards-based teaching techniques, approaches, and concepts that may be interesting to teachers throughout the state. The final issue of linking the informal community of teachers with the formal teacher education system administered by the university is inherent again in the fact that this is a university project. Teachers will be able to seek advice from professors who are online in the community. Some university instructors are already using the pilot site as a part of their pre-service teacher education courses, and plans are in the works to use an area of the site for distance education courses.

Finally, the element of fostering ownership and participation is experienced through the fact that the site is managed by the teacher participants themselves and only administered by the university. One pitfall of traditional teacher development is minimized. Participants engage in self-exploration and an opportunity to share and build a community. The asynchronous communication within the site allows teachers to enter the site at their own convenience and meet their own needs. Also, they can reflect on their own practice and work with others who can add to the depth of that reflection.

CONCLUSIONS AND IMPLICATIONS

The iteration of the ILF is but a first attempt to create a professional development community situated in real practice and delivered via the WWW. To accomplish this task, we combined the best of virtual teacher development models, used video to situate practices, and are collaborating with practicing teachers to create their community of practice. In this manner, we have incorporated the theory and principles discussed to create online professional development for pre-service and in-service teachers.

The ILF prototype presents numerous unanswered questions for future research: What factors underlie the effective use of electronic technologies to foster, sustain, and scale a virtual community? What principles enable a community of practice to value sharing of practice and dialogue in such ways as to outweigh participation costs–time, technology access, and the sacrifice of ego attached to one's teaching? How do people learn in and from the ILF, and how is that learning reflected in the classroom? How do the ILF members structure themselves into communities and how do we promote boundary crossing? How does the group transmit to newcomers the skills, knowledge, and values that constitute being an effective teacher? The ILF research team will continue to examine and explore these issues and look forward to enhancing the understanding of professional development in higher education on the World Wide Web. Currently, Barab and colleagues have received a National Science Foundation grant for $1.5 million to grow and do research on the ILF (see the current site at *http://ilf.crlt.indiana. edu*).

Darling-Hammond (1993) reminds us that the new school reform paradigm starts with the assumption that students are not standardized and that teaching is not routine. We believe that this fact holds true for professional development as well. Growth and development for teachers is not routine and should not be made uniform. Likewise, the ILF is hardly routine, and we look at it as only a beginning. We eagerly anticipate the comments of teacher participants and readers to guide us in enriching the project as we all develop our professional teaching community into the 21st century, and to continue to explore many of the unanswered questions and pose new ones as the community grows over the life of the project.

AUTHORS' NOTE

The authors are indebted to the efforts of the members of Education R685–Professional Development for the 21st Century class at Indiana University, Spring 1999: Faculty: Bob Appelman, Sasha Barab, Tom Duffy, Enrique Galindo, Tom Keating, and Mary McMullen; Students: Michael Barnett, Brian Beatty, Chin-Chi Chao, Kursat Cagalitay, Judy East, Heredina Galindo, Jamie Kirkley, Judith Longfield, Jim MacKinster, Julie Moore, Jeff Nowak, Diana Treahy, Eric Reynolds, and Ji Yoon Yoon; Anchor Teachers: Jill Fabiano, Rise Paynter, Nancy Stockwell, Wendy Tamborrino in the design and implementation of the ILF prototype.

REFERENCES

Ball, D. (1996). Teacher learning and the mathematics reforms: What we think we know and what we need to know. *Phi Delta Kappan, 77*, 500-08.

Barab, S. A., & Duffy, T. (2000). From practice fields to communities of practice. In D. Jonassen, & S. M. Land (Eds.). *Theoretical foundations of learning environments* (pp. 25-56). Mahwah, NJ: Lawrence Erlbaum.

Barab, S. A., Cherkes-Julkowski, M., Swenson, R., Garrett. S., Shaw, R. E., & Young, M. E. (1999). Principles of self-organization: Ecologizing the learner-facilitator system. *Journal of the Learning Sciences*.

Barab, S. A., Squire, K., & Dueber, W. (2000). A co-evolutionary model for supporting the emergence of authenticity. *Educational Technology Research and Development, 48*(2), 37-62.

Brown, J. S., Collins, A., & Duguid, P. (1989). Situated cognition and the culture of learning. *Educational Researcher, 18*, 32-42.

Brown, J. S., & Duguid, P. (1998). Organizing knowledge. *California Management Review, 40*, 90-111.

Chaney, T. (1995). *Design and implementation of a constructivist instructional model to support teacher change: A case study.* Unpublished dissertation study. Bloomington, IN: Indiana University.

Chaney-Cullen, T., & Duffy, T. (1998) Strategic teaching frameworks: Multimedia to support teacher change. *Journal of the Learning Sciences, 8*, 1-40.

Chism, N. (1985). *The place of peer interaction in teacher development: Findings from a case study.* Paper presented at the Annual Meeting of the American Educational Research Association (Chicago, IL, March 31-April 4, 1985). ERIC database access number: ED262469.

Darling-Hammond (1993). Reframing the school reform agenda. *Phi Delta Kappan*, *74*, 752-61.

Darling-Hammond, L. (1996). The quiet revolution: Rethinking teacher development. *Educational Leadership*, *53*(6), 4-10.

Duffy, Thomas M. (1997). Strategic teaching framework: An instructional model for a constructivist learning environment. In C. Dills & A. Romiszowski (Eds.), *Instructional development state of the art. Volume 3: Paradigms*. Englewood, NJ: Educational Technology Press.

Greeno, J. G. (1998). The situativity of knowing, learning, and research. *American Psychologist*, *53*, 5-26.

Indiana Professional Standards Board (1996). *Draft standards for teachers of mathematics*. Indianapolis, IN: Indiana Professional Standards Board.

Interstate New Teacher Assessment and Support Consortium (1991). *Model standards for beginning teacher licensing and development: A resource for state dialogue* (Working Draft). Washington, DC: Council of Chief State of School Officers.

Lagache, E. (1993). *"Diving" into communities of practice: Examining learning as legitimate peripheral participation in an everyday setting*. Paper presented at the Annual Meeting of the American Educational Research Association (Atlanta, GA, April 12-16, 1993). ERIC database access number: ED360387.

Lambdin, D., Duffy, T., & Moore, J. (1997). Using an information system to expand preservice teachers' visions of effective mathematics teaching. *Journal of Technology and Teacher Education*, *5*, 171-202.

Lave, J. (1993). Introduction. In J. Lave & S. Chaiklin (Eds.), *Understanding practice: Perspectives on activity and context* (pp. 3-34). New York: Cambridge University Press.

Lave, J., & Wenger, E. (1991). *Situated learning: Legitimate peripheral participation*. New York: Cambridge University Press.

Reynolds, E., & O'Neil, M. (1997). Exploring teacher education through video. In S. Cornwell, P. Rule, & T. Sugino (Eds.), *Proceedings of the Annual JALT International Conference on Language Teaching and Learning* (23rd, Hiroshima, Japan, November 1996), 48-52.

Ruopp, R., Gal, S., Drayton, B., & Pfister, M. (Eds.) (1993). *LabNet: Toward a community of practice*. Hillsdale, NJ: Lawrence Erlbaum.

Seely-Brown, J. (1998). Internet technology in support of the concept of "communities of practice": The case of Xerox. *Accounting Management and Information Technologies*, *8*, 227-236.

Smylie, M. A., & Conyers, J. G. (1991). Changing conceptions of teaching influence: The future of staff development. *Journal of Staff Development*, *12*(1), 12-16.

Willis, E. M. (1997). Technology: Integrated into, not added onto, the curriculum experiences in pre-service teacher education. *Computers in the Schools*, *13*(1/2), 141-153.

Wim de Boer
Betty Collis

Implementation and Adaptation Experiences with a WWW-Based Course Management System

SUMMARY. Members of the faculty of educational science and technology of the University of Twente, The Netherlands, have been making innovative use of WWW-based course-support sites since 1994. By 2000 all of the faculty were involved not only in using the WWW, but also more fundamentally in a new educational approach. In addition, our educational technologists collaborate with other faculties to support the same progression. How has this come about? In this article, the *TeleTOP Method (http://teletop.edte.utwente.nl)* is described, showing how it has developed based on an implementation model and experience acquired with innovative use of the WWW for course support. The applicability of the model to other faculties and settings is discussed. *[Article copies available for a fee from The Haworth Document Delivery Service: 1-800-342-9678. E-mail address: <getinfo@haworthpressinc.com> Website: <http://www.HaworthPress. com> © 2001 by The Haworth Press, Inc. All rights reserved.]*

KEYWORDS. WWW-based course-management system, implementation, adaptation, uses of a WWW system

WIM DE BOER is Educational Designer on the TeleTOP Team, Faculty of Educational Science and Technology, University of Twente, P.O. Box 217, Enschede, The Netherlands (E-mail: w.f.deboer@edte.utwente.nl).
BETTY COLLIS is Professor, Faculty of Educational Science and Technology, University of Twente, P.O. Box 217, Enschede, The Netherlands (E-mail: collis@ edte.utwente.nl).

[Haworth co-indexing entry note]: "Implementation and Adaptation Experiences with a WWW-Based Course Management System." de Boer, Wim. and Betty Collis. Co-published simultaneously in *Computers in the Schools* (The Haworth Press. Inc.) Vol. 17. No. 3/4, 2001. pp. 127-146; and: *The Web in Higher Education: Assessing the Impact and Fulfilling the Potential* (ed: Cleborne D. Maddux, and D. LaMont Johnson) The Haworth Press, Inc., 2001, pp. 127-146. Single or multiple copies of this article are available for a fee from The Haworth Document Delivery Service [1-800-342-9678, 9:00 a.m. - 5:00 p.m. (EST). E-mail address: getinfo@haworthpressinc.com].

127

At the University of Twente "tele-learning," or the application of information and communication technology to support our teaching and learning processes, has a high priority (Collis, 1998a). In our use of the term, tele-learning does not necessarily imply distance education. Instead it emphasizes the increased flexibility that can come to the teaching and learning process through the combination of the new possibilities offered by the World Wide Web (WWW) and new ways of teaching and learning. The most ambitious of the tele-learning initiatives at the University of Twente is the *TeleTOP* project of the faculty of Educational Science and Technology. The overall goal of the TeleTOP initiative is to encourage the innovative and appropriate use of the WWW for learning purposes within the faculty in order to enhance educational delivery and make it more efficient and more flexible. The core ideas of TeleTOP are extending the levels of activity and engagement of students and extending the impact and influence of instructors (Collis, 1998b). At the same time, this is a pioneering approach to the education of both regular students and mature students who remain in their homes and jobs while they participate in the program. This new approach, *C@mpus+*, extends the benefits of the campus experience to both regular and distance students.

To support this new approach, we identified core requirements for a WWW-based course-management system (Tielemans & Collis, 1999) by capitalizing on our own experiences. In 1997 we built our own system, based upon a Lotus Notes database. Instructors and students do not have any contact with Notes clients; it is a key requirement that both instructors and students are able to work with the system through any simple HTML browser (such as Netscape) and on any compuer, as long as it is connected to the Internet. However, no matter how elegant a system is, instructors must use it, an administration must choose to support its use and thus must make resources available, the technical infrastructure already in place must handle it, and software and hardware must be available.

The decision made by the faculty of Educational Science and Technology in 1997 was to redesign all courses, both pedagogically and including use of WWW tools and environments. This involved the challenge of working with a wide variety of courses and instructors. We began by redesigning all the first-year couses, then all the second-year courses. By the end of the year 2000 we had redesigned all the other courses. (See *http://teletop.edte.utwente.nl*, through which a number of courses can be visited for inspection and many publications and presentations are available.) We also have responded to other faculties who wanted to make use of our system and methodology. The first was the faculty of Telematics, a technical faculty in our own university with many engineering and mathematics courses. The adaptation proceeded smoothly, and has moved to the rest of the faculties in the university, as well as faculties in other universities.

In this article, we describe the TeleTOP Implementation Model that delineates, based on the literature and our experiences, the change entities that are of importance when an institution plans to implement the WWW in education on a wide scale. We also describe the adaptation process for the Telematics faculty. The questions addressed by this article are:

1. What factors influence the initiation, implementation, and institutionalization phases of using a WWW-based course-management system to fundamentally change teaching and learning?
2. Can the TeleTOP Implementation Model assist faculties other than the one for which it was developed in these change phases?

DEVELOPING THE IMPLEMENTATION MODEL

An educational change never concerns one entity (i.e., a WWW-based course-management system). It always involves more than one aspect. Fullan (1991) notes that an educational change involves the materials used for instruction, the instructional approaches, and the pedagogical convictions of those involved. Ideally, the change should become institutionalized in all three of these aspects. However, what is often the case is that an instructor may only change in one or two of these aspects–using a WWW site, for example, but not changing his or her instructional approach or view of what comprises good teaching and course delivery. Unfortunately, while institutionalization with respect to computer technology, and now network technology, has generally occurred at the materials (in terms of technical infrastructure) level in higher education, institutionalization of changed instructional methods and changed pedagogical convictions has not yet passed through the implementation phase (and in many institutions, has not even begun the initiation phase). For confirmation of this, see a recent study commissioned by the Ministry of Education in The Netherlands that reviewed the use of ICT in higher education internationally (Collis & Wende, 1999). Clearly the change process is still not well enough understood, or those responsible for the change process have difficulty translating their understandings into practice, or both. There is a need for an implementation model that not only describes the change process but also can serve as a guide for those involved in each phase of the process. Thus we developed the TeleTOP Implementation Model initially to guide our own work and then, to be a tool for other faculties. The model involves two sets of variables related to time and to change entities.

Changes Related to Time

Change processes in educational organizations have been extensively studied (Fullan, 1991; Plomp, 1992). There is general agreement that three phases of change over time can be identified. Typically, these are called an initiation phase, an implementation phase, and an institutionalization phase (Fullan, 1991). The initiation phase involves many processes and dynamics that lead to the decision that a certain change target is chosen and a change process started. After the change is initiated, the implementation phase evolves, often as a series of experiments tested in practice relating to the change target. In the institutional phase, the change is no longer at the experimental level but is integrated into the institution's regular operations. The transition from initiation through implementation to institutionalization with a technological innovation in higher education can be expected to be at least a five-year process (Plomp, 1992). Thus, overall success cannot be expected quickly.

Although the implementation phase is only one of the three phases in the change process related to time, the entire process is often called an implementation process. Also, the linearity of the process is not as direct as these three phases would indicate. Within any innovation, there will be many sub-innovations, some of which will only be at the initiation phase while others may be in the institutionalization phase. The success of early sub-innovations (success being defined as institutionalization) can be taken as a partial indicator of the likelihood of the full change being successful. Conversely, the lack of success of early sub-innovations should be taken as a warning. The initiation phase has a major effect on what follows, and thus, the factors that influence an organization to commit itself to start a change process or not are of particular importance. Thus, one dimension of the TeleTOP Implementation Model for a WWW-based course-management system in a faculty is that of time, expressed in terms of Fullan's three phases of initiation, implementation, and institutionalization.

Change Entities

While the change phases provide a dimension for studying the change process relating to a technological innovation in an educational institution, what makes the change process concrete are entities that relate specifically to what happens in practice. These change entities also change in their importance to the overall process over time. Twelve change entities have emerged from the first three years of the TeleTOP experience and the continual literature analysis that has occurred. These entities have their major impact during a particular phase of the overall change process, but that does not mean that they are not important in the other phases as well. Figure 1 shows the TeleTOP Implementation Model. Following the Figure, the 12 change entities are briefly described.

1. Both Plomp (1992) and Fullan (1991) note that the *educational target* is an important change entity. It has four different characteristics: relevance, clarity, complexity, and quality. With respect to relevance and clarity, it is important that those involved with the change know what the goals of the change are and also recognize the importance of the change. With a WWW-based course-management system, this means clarity in understanding what such a system is and acceptance of the relevance of the system for the institution. The target purpose for the use of a WWW-based course- management system will vary from institution to institution. With TeleTOP, for example, the target was to enable the *C@mpus+* approach, whereby mature students primarily at a distance can participate equally and fully with on-campus students in course activities. The third characteristic of the entity relates to the complexity of the change. Rosenblum and Louis (1981) have found somewhat paradoxically that complex changes are more often successful than simple changes when appropriate methodologies are used in all phases of the change process. This relates to the characteristic of quality.

2. The institutional administration is a critical factor in the likelihood that appropriate methodologies will be carried out (Berman & McLaughlin, 1977). In the initiation phase, the administration has the role of setting up and funding the initiation processes. The administration must also have an active role in the implementation phase. One such aspect is financial support of faculty workshops and other forms of training. The administration must also acknowledge that change will take time and will require financing through this time. All of these are reflected in the change entity *budget*.

3. Another change entity is the receptivity of the organization to change and innovation. This in turn relates to the extent that other sorts of innovative activities have been rewarded and valued in the past. Berman and McLaughlin note that earlier positive experiences with change processes are likely to be correlated with a positive attitude

among those in the organization to a new change process. An *innovative culture* is thus another change entity.

4. The basic style of the change process can be one where the administration initiates change or one where changes grow as a result of interest and pressure from instructors or students. Both directions of pressure for change have their important aspects and probably both are needed in some form of balance. Thus, another entity in the change process is expressed as *bottom-up or top-down*, but should be a combination of both.

5. The fourth aspect that Plomp mentioned as critical to the change process in an organization was quality of the educational target. Quality relates to more than only the educational target, it also relates to the technologies involved in the change process. Quality is necessary in order that instructors are attracted to technologies. Quality also affects the level of confidence that the instructors have about the technologies. They need to know that the technologies have been tested in practice, are reliable and easy to use, easy to understand in terms of use, and practical. The not-invented-here feeling can sometimes make instructors skeptical about a technology product purchased from an outside source. On the other hand, instructors may also wonder about the robustness of systems developed in-house. Two entities in the model relate to these quality aspects. The first relates to the origin of the software to be used–*Software that is bought or built*. The second relates to the technical infrastructure that will support the innovation–*Quality hardware and network*.

6. In the specific case of WWW-based course-management systems, it is preferable that the system should support the existing ways of teaching in an organization in order to get instructors over the threshold for use. However, the same system should also facilitate courses to become more enriched, more flexible, and more efficient (Collis, 1998b) in a way that seems a comfortable growth process for the instructor. Learning to work with the WWW-based system should not take instructors much time, and the system should be easy to integrate into their existing ways of working. It is important that the system can adapt to the way that an individual instructor wants to work, even as the instructor, too, will need to make some adaptation in his or her typical teaching practices. The extent to which it takes the instructor time and energy to make the change (i.e., to learn how to use the course-management system) is a useful index for the amount of resistance that will occur to the change (House, 1974). *Fit with instructional practices* is therefore an important change entity, directly related to the educational target. The

instructor's perceptions of the quality of the system based on his or her own experience and that of immediate peers will have a larger influence than objective criteria on the likelihood of the instructor's acceptance of the system (Van der Veen & De Boer, 1999). How well the instructor perceives that the course management system fits his or her established instructional practices is a major determinant of the instructor's subjective reactions.

7. The *initiation target* that started the change process is also an interesting change entity. The initiation target is different from the education target when it focuses on a strategic goal such as gaining more students. An initiation target must be convincing in terms of its payoff to the institution.

8. In the initiation phase, certain persons start certain processes so that the organization starts thinking about the change. The persons who can start this process could be members of the administration, but also could be individual instructors. If instructors, they are, in general, enthusiastic. However, it is not always the case that the pioneers have a position in the institution that gives weight and audience to their ideas. *Key figures to initiate* therefore is an important change entity because the key figures must make clear the goal of the change (important, according to Plomp and Fullan) and must influence the climate for change. They are also the persons who could initiate the sub-innovation of a social-learning environment in the institution, stimulating colleagues to benefit from the experiences of each other (Fullan, 1991).

9. To successfully move from the initiation phase to the implementation phase, some entities that were important in the initiation phase must remain important while others will fade. Those that remain important include: the educational target remains clear, the technologies (in this case, the WWW-based system and tools) remain easy to use and are perceived as practical to the instructors, and the administration remains publicly committed to the change. Visscher (1996) indicates that a technological system should have a high success factor in its early usage, for example, an instructor should be able to get started quickly and successfully with a small and orderly part of the WWW-based system. For this quick start to occur and for a community of practice to begin to develop where the users of the system can benefit from each other's experiences, a *Project Team* needs to be formed. The team must function well, working both responsively and proactively to coordinate and lead the ongoing activities.

10. When, after a few successful years, the administration decides to migrate the change into the normal ongoing practices in the institution,

the change is in fact no longer a change but has been institutionalized. In this phase, where *Embedding of Use* is occurring, a *Structural Support Group* needs to support the normal use of the system. Usually this will be the existing technical or educational-support group in the institution. It is challenging when some aspects of a change process are at the institutionalization phase and thus require the help of the structural support group, and others are still at the implementation phase requiring the Project Team, or even at the initiation phase requiring the intervention of key figures. In these cases, the same team and leadership might be expected to fulfill roles with different demands and requiring different skills (Collis & Moonen, 1994). This complexity may be one of the major challenges in the overall change process.

While the model helps us understand our own experiences, to what extent does it generalize to help another faculty?

ADAPTATION EXPERIENCES

In January 1999 it was decided that the new Telematics faculty at the University of Twente should also set up a WWW-based course-support environment as had been done at the faculty of Educational Science and Technology. A project group was set up which would be responsible for the technical and instructional implementation of TeleTOP in this new faculty. A key question was if the educational culture and approach in one faculty could map on to that in another faculty. The project group consisted of two TeleTOP team members and two members of the Telematics faculty. The Telematics members were primarily responsible for the implementation while the transfer of the TeleTOP method and course-management system was the responsibility of the TeleTOP team members.

Figure 2 gives an impression of how the TeleTOP team planned the steps for the transfer and adaptation of TeleTOP to another faculty (a process repeated in March-June 1999 for a faculty in another university). Figure 2 is an operational version of the TeleTOP Implementation Model shown in Figure 1.

The actual implementation steps visualized in Figure 2 are summarized in the following sections. Comments are provided as to what was intended in the steps, and what actually occurred in the transfer process.

1. Defining the target group, context, goals and making a plan. These activities relate to the first steps in the initiation phase of the TeleTOP Implementation Model. The groups involved should be identified, the

FIGURE 1. The TeleTOP Implementation Model, Version 1

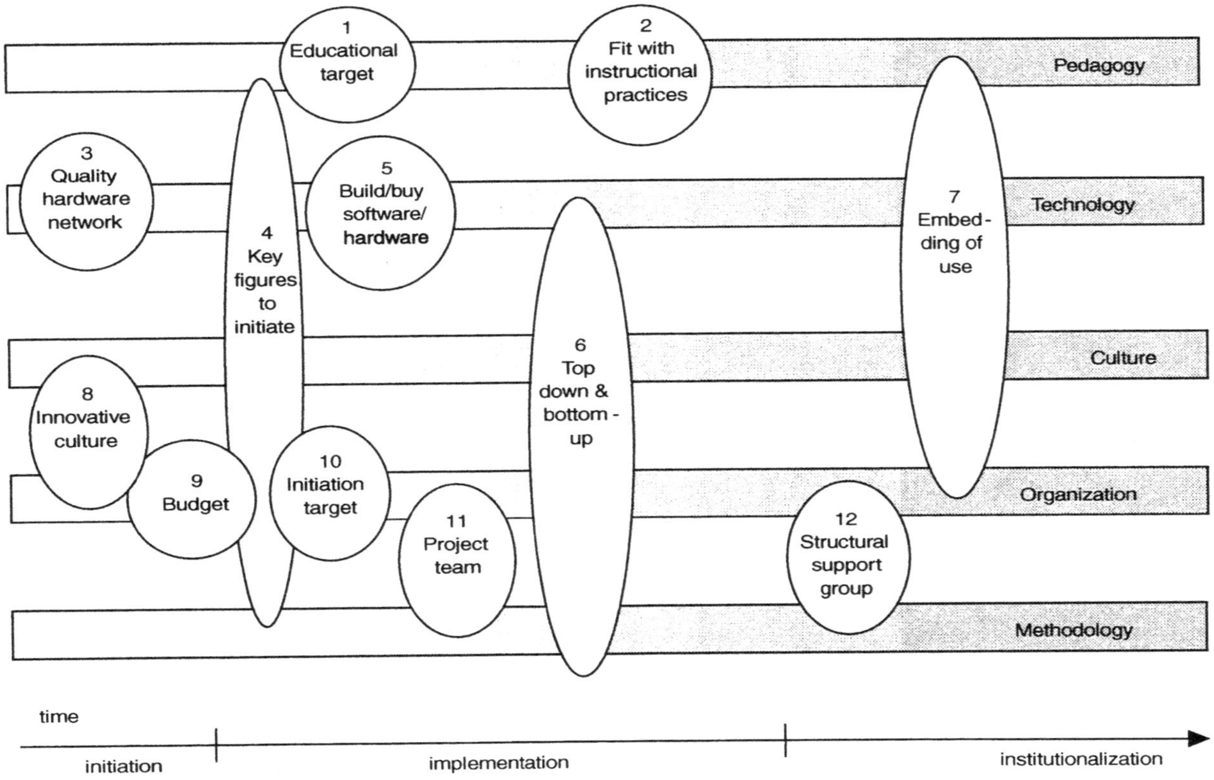

Pedagogy

Technology

Culture

Organization

Methodology

1 Educational target

2 Fit with instructional practices

3 Quality hardware network

4 Key figures to initiate

5 Build/buy software/ hardware

6 Top down & bottom - up

7 Embed- ding of use

8 Innovative culture

9 Budget

10 Initiation target

11 Project team

12 Structural support group

time

initiation

implementation

institutionalization

135

technical infrastructure should be made clear, as well as the skills of the persons involved: instructors, technical people, and educational-support staff. In the planning, the goal of the innovation chosen, and which financial and human resources would make it all possible must be clarified. In the Telematics-faculty situation, while most of these activities occurred, the goal of the innovation was not made explicitly clear to all involved. The Telematics faculty coordinator planned a start-up session with all who were involved at the beginning of the project, and indicated that the initiative was very important with regards to providing more flexibility for the students. No specific educational targets were mentioned. The commitment of the faculty management was evident because extra money and resources were made available. The planning should indicate when the course-management system should be operational for use. This occurred, as the Telematics faculty chose to start the actual work in March 1999, with the first three courses running at the start of the new academic year, in September 1999. However, before the actual use of the system there would be two trials. Thus, the first step of the adaptation process proceeded generally as planned, but in an uneven way. Planning and selection of target group was well handled, but setting of goals was only at an abstract level. Perhaps because of the culture and context in the faculty (a desire to be seen as innovative users of telematics technology and a high comfort level with technology use in general), the first step in the adaptation process nonetheless moved smoothly within the Telematics faculty. In other faculties without this culture, technical comfort level and underlying motivation for change, the goals of the innovation would have to be argued more explicitly.

FIGURE 2. Steps for Adapting the TeleTOP Implementation Model and Methodology to Another Faculty

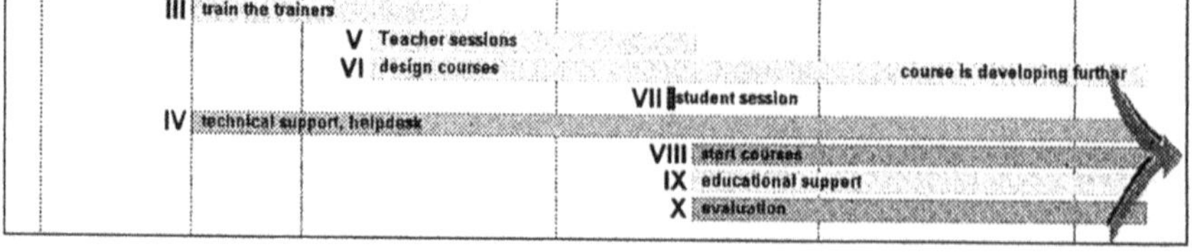

II. Set up the technical infrastructure. The operational model shown in Figure 2 indicates that the technical infrastructure for the WWW-based course-management system should be set up in Months 2 and 3. In the case of the Telematics faculty, this was not a problem. There was already a sophisticated technical infrastructure existing with the faculty, an excellent network in place, and multi-media computers for all students and staff. Therefore the only requirements were to set up a Lotus Notes Domino server and to guide the faculty Web masters in learning some new skills for maintaining it. In faculties without highly skilled technical staff, this second step could take much longer.

III. & IV. Train the trainers and technical support, helpdesk. It was decided that the instructors in the Telematics faculty should have easy access to educational and technical support. Therefore the support group should be physically close at hand. The person responsible for educational support already had general experience in helping the instructors and thus only needed to be educated in using the new software for different kinds of learning situations. The educational-support person also learned to work with the TeleTOP tools that support different types of learning activities and to get hands-on experience. This step of the adaptation went smoothly.

V & VI. Instructor sessions and designing the course. The next step was to set up a series of sessions for the telematics instructors. The topics dealt with in the sessions were technical as well as instructional. After the first session, during which members of the administration introduced their plans, a technical session followed. The course-management system was demonstrated and instructors had the chance to try it out themselves. Two weeks later a personal session was arranged. In a one-hour interview, the educational support-group member showed the instructor examples of how the WWW could be used in support of technical courses, trying to get a first indication of what would suit the particular course and wishes of the instructor. After this, every other week a two-hour hands-on session was held. Instructors used the management environments for their own courses, to try things out and to exchange ideas. Most instructors attended these meetings and thought they were worthwhile. The instructors used their time getting skilled in using the course-management system while at the same time designing their own courses. It must be noted that most course-redesign work was put off until only a few weeks before the starting date of a course. Nonetheless, Steps V and VI went as planned. Figure 3 is a screen dump of the WWW-environment used to support the instructor sessions.

VII. Student session. The use of the TeleTOP course support-management system proved to be a very user-friendly system for the students (based on the results of a student evaluation; Fisser, Van de Kamp, & Slot, 1999). Students learned the basics and were able to work with the system within one short session. All students received a basic manual. They learned more about additional features of the environments as they used them during their courses. Thus Step VII also went as planned.

VIII & IX. Start the courses and educational support. The courses could start after the student session, and after the students had gotten access to the course-management environments. The use of the TeleTOP system made it possible to have a variety of forms of interactions within the environment, and to let the environment "grow" during the time the course was held. During the time that the courses were in operation, ed-

FIGURE 3. Screen Capture of the TeleTOP Site Supporting Group and Personal Sessions with Instructors

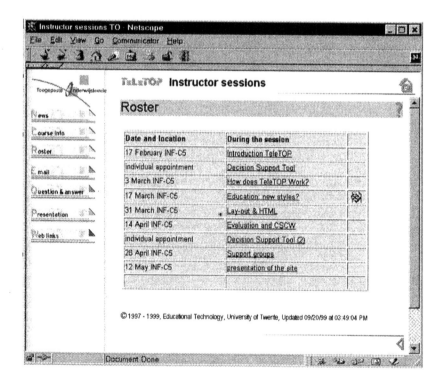

ucational support was available to the instructors, as well as technical support (see Step IV). Most instructors, however, were capable of managing their own environments. Thus Steps VIII and IX proceeded smoothly and as planned.

X. Evaluation. The key evaluation question was: Can a method and system developed to reflect the educational culture and approach in one faculty map on to that in another faculty? A special evaluation team was set up to provide an answer to this and other questions. The main outcomes of the evaluation (Fisser, Van de Kamp, & Slot, 1999) were:

1. The transfer process was carried out to the satisfaction of the Telematics faculty, and within a limited amount of time investment by the TeleTOP team.
2. The personal sessions between the administrator and the instructors were experienced as valuable.
3. Most instructors were well informed about the developments about TeleTOP from the start of the implementation, but some instructors experienced a lack of clarity concerning the goal(s) of the educational change.
4. Instructors have enough technical skills to use the environment in their courses. They are positive about the instructor sessions, but would like to have a more specific manual.
5. The frequency of interaction between instructors and students has become higher. The management should take into account the extra effort.
6. Students are positive about the flexibility of the change, but they have some concerns about becoming too dependent on a technical system in case of technical failure, and the costs.

Summarizing the evaluation, the TeleTOP Implementation Model did seem to describe reasonably the experiences of the Telematics faculty in initiating and implementing the use of a WWW-based course-management system. The Model also served as a basis for planning of the initiation and implementation phases. Thus the TeleTOP Implementation Model did seem to describe reasonably the experiences of the Telematics faculty as it had earlier described the experiences of the faculty of Educational Science and Technology. However, the model does not explicitly focus on what happens in the teaching and learning process. What sorts of teaching and learning experiences took place in the two faculties? Were they also similar?

DIFFERENCES IN THE USE OF A WWW-BASED
COURSE MANAGEMENT

Since 1997, courses have been using the TeleTOP system at the faculty of Educational Science and Technology. The faculty of Telematics in contrast had only been using the system since early 1999. Thus differences in use could reflect the amount of experience or the nature of the faculty (technical or social science) or both. Evaluations carried out in 1999 in both faculties (Bloemen, 1999; Fisser, Van de Kamp, & Slot, 1999) studied the instructional uses of the TeleTOP system with a particular interest in comparing the choices instructors made about the different tools they would use within their course environments.

Both groups of instructors were unanimous about three features in the system: (a) the News feature whereby an instructor can easily post general messages to the student, (b) the Course Information feature whereby instructors have templates in which they enter standard course information such as course objectives and evaluation criteria, and (c) a WWW-based matrix (which we call a *roster*) as an organizing structure for course content, activities, communication, and feedback. The course-information templates were appreciated, as their contents could immediately be used by the faculty administration for the printed course guides as well as the faculty's informational WWW pages. The roster relates more directly to the instructional approach that the instructor chooses for a course. For example, the instructor is free to choose the number of rows and columns for the matrix and organize them in any way he or she wishes. This includes having views associated with each of the cells in the matrix that may contain student work and communication, as well as instructor feedback. Figure 4 shows samples of the options that were chosen by the instructors of 26 courses of Educational Science and Technology, and 10 instructors of the Faculty of Telematics.

As comparisons of how instructors chose to design and use their rosters, Figure 5 shows the roster of *TeleLearning*, a course of the faculty of Educational Science and Technology. The roster in the *TeleLearning* course gives an overview of the assignments and meetings of the course. The course was organized around contact sessions. Instead of lectures, the students present on campus could interact with each other in a variety of ways, while students not present could participate, within 48 hours, via the course site on the WWW. For students not able to participate as part of the real-time group during any of the sessions, participation in the group session was also expected, but asynchronously and via the WWW.

FIGURE 4. Percentages of Instructors Using Various Options in TeleTOP (for Educational Science & Technology, $N = 26$, and for Telematics, $N = 10$; First Half 1999)

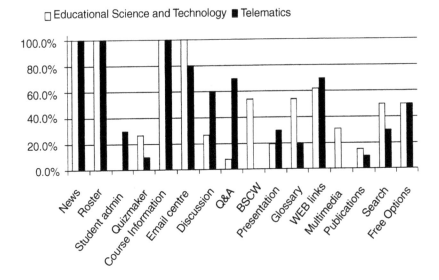

A major aspect of the instructional approach of the course was the ability for students to work in groups on a design and development project that could be linked to the WWW site in a shared workspace (called BSCW), and later in the Presentation Area of the site so that all students could study each other's work and give peer feedback.

Figure 6 shows the roster of *Switching and Control Systems*, a course given at the faculty of Telematics. In this course, students were accountable for presenting more than half the lectures. Students formed groups and chose a topic about which they were to present material to their fellow students and the instructors. All materials were placed in the session row of the roster of that particular week. The first part of the lecture session was the actual lecture; the second part was intended for questions and discussions. Also, after the sessions, the discussion would continue in the discussion area of the site. The site was therefore intended as a real support site, to be used for information, student- and instructor-contributed materials, and communication.

FIGURE 5. The Roster of the Course *Tele-learning* (Educational Science and Technology Faculty)

Roster			
Before the session	Date and location	During the session	After the session
	23 March 99, L209 (IAC), 8:30-10:25	Intro to course; Intro to video in WWW sites; guest Mr Jose Bidarra	Find & reflect: Example of educational WWW site with video (5 pts)
Read Chs 1 & 2. Submit follow-up questions (5 pts)	30 March 99, L209	Extending the lecture, Guest visitor (dr. S. Santema)	Evaluate two examples of the extended lecture (5 pts)
Read Ch.6: (Submit response: 5 pts, due 5-4-99)	6 April 99, 8:30, L209	Introducing the project. Using the template, choosing roles; Intro to the videoconference the next week	Content: HTML, Video, and teams meet. Manager reports (by 21:00 Sunday 11 April, 5 points)
read Ch 4: No written assignment but click to get more information...	13 April, 8:30, L209, & 15 April, videoconference (15:30-17:00)	General comments on planning, group work; Differences to note between the video conf & asynchronous settings	Comments about the videoconference (25 April 10 pts)
	20 April, L209, 8:30-10:25	Walkthrough, video plans;	Self-evaluation comments (5 pts)
Read Ch. 8, respond to questions (5 pts)	27 April, L209, 8:30-10:25	Design principles for WWW sites with video	Apply design principles to an external site (9 May, 10 pts)
	18 May	Issues confronting the use of the WWW (with & without video) in education	Finish your group projects. Due, for evaluation; 20 May 1999
Read Ch 10	25 May, L209, 8:30-10:25	Present group projects (video captured), (30 pts)	Reflection on the course, and on tele-learning (15 pts)

Looking at Figure 4 and taking into account the two examples of the use of the roster shown in Figures 5 and 6, it can be concluded that the differences in use of the TeleTOP system between the two faculties were not very large. It seems that the faculty of Telematics focuses a little more on communication via the support environment, and the faculty of Educational Science and Technology focuses more on collaborative work through the support environment. However, as the examples in Figures 5 and 6 show, both aspects appear in the WWW environments of both faculties. The Telematics faculty was still at the beginning of the implementation phase, and had a long way to go until full institutionalization. It will be interesting to follow the faculties and see where they will be in one or two years (De Boer & Collis, 2000; Messing & Collis, 2000). Maybe the differences will fade away or maybe they will increase.

FIGURE 6. The Roster of the Course *Switches and Control Systems* (Telematics faculty)

Roster				?
Before the session	**Date and location**	**During the session**	**After the session**	
Register with BOOZ EL	Mon 22 March, 5/6th, hour, CT1845	Introduction	Form groups	
	26 March	No Lecture on this day.		
D1. Docent- Lecture.	Fri 9 April, 5/6th hour BB109	Introduction to Wide Area networks.		
D2. Read performance analysis material in the reader. Docent-Lecture.	Fri 16 April, 5/6th hour BB109	Performance Analysis Background	Assignment D2 available 24 April, and due 10 May 12.00.	
S1. Read material in the reader. Group S1 prepares the lecture. Group S6 prepares the questions.	Mon 19 April, 5/6th hour ELTN10152	Architecture of Switches and Routers		
S2. Read material in the reader. Group S2 prepares the lecture. Group S7 prepares the questions.	Fri 23 April, 5/6th hour BB109	Performance Analysis of Switches.		
	7 May	No lecture on this day.	Assignment D2 worked out.	
S3. Read material in the reader. Group S3 prepares the lecture. Group S1 prepares the questions	Mon 17 May, 5/6th hour ELTN10152	Signalling Systems.		
S4. Read material in the reader. Group S4 prepares the lecture. Group S5 prepares the questions.	Fri 21 May, 5/6th hour ELTN10152	IP over ATM		
D3. Read material in the reader on MPLS and IP Switching. Docent- Lecture.	Fri 28 May, 5/6th hour ELTN10152	IP Switching	Assignment D3 is available. Due in one week on 4 June 1999	

CONCLUSION

The questions studied were:

1. What is a model that describes the factors that influence a faculty during the initiation, implementation, and institutionalization phases of the use of a WWW-based course-management system for fundamental changes in its ways of teaching and learning?
2. Does the TeleTOP Implementation Model assist faculties other than the one for which it was developed in these change phases?

The TeleTOP Implementation Model is our response to the first question. The comparison between the more theoretical model and the practical steps taken with the Telematics faculty shows that the model generally fits the practice in this particular case. In a subsequent study of ten other faculties or universities, the TeleTOP Implementation Model was also found to be a good fit for describing what had gone on within those institutions (De Boer & Collis, 1999). In terms of the second question, the model identified a series of steps that were used to guide the initiation and implementation processes for the Telematics faculty as it got ready for the use of the TeleTOP WWW-based course-management system to support its courses. It is, however, a question as to whether the implementation could be even more successful if the model had been used before the actual change was started. An important step, according to the TeleTOP Implementation Model, was to clarify the goal of the change. In the case of the Telematics faculty, this entity was not given that much thought. Would the instructors be more committed if the administration addressed more attention to this matter? Or was the implicit motivation of being involved in a state-of-the-art use of a telematics application enough to motivate this young faculty, anxious to be seen as offering top-level education, and practicing what it preaches in terms of making use of telematics? It may also have been the case that the experiences of the Educational Science and Technology faculty had to serve a pioneer function and thus more care was needed on the rationale for use of a WWW-based system than was the case on a faculty that started later and could already see that one faculty was proceeding smoothly.

In general, the TeleTOP Implementation Model seems to indicate a number of factors that influence the implementation of an educational and organizational change such as the use of the WWW within a faculty, and seems to be helpful in guiding this change. The model is being used to steer a number of other adaptation experiences, as well as continued work within its home faculty. The model appears to be a valuable aid for a faculty to help it keep the many different aspects relating to the successful initiation, implementation, and institutionalization of a WWW-based course-management system in focus and balance. Too often, the dominant attention seems to be given to the choice of technical platform; a model can show that the technical platform is just one of many factors that need careful attention.

AUTHORS' NOTE

Dr. Wim de Boer is an educational designer on the TeleTOP team and also working on his PhD where his topic is the validation of the TeleTOP Implementation Model. He has recently participated in a national study whose aim was to develop an evaluation framework for WWW-based course-management systems.

Dr. Betty Collis is Professor of Tele-Learning at the University of Twente in The Netherlands and also Senior Researcher, Advanced Learning Technologies, at the multi-faculty research institute CTIT at the same institution. She is also chair of the TeleTOP Initiative. She is a pioneer in the use of the WWW in teaching, since March 1994, using the WWW with all of her own courses. For more information, see: http://users.edte.utwente.nl/collis/

REFERENCES

Berman, P., & McLaughlin, M. W. (1977). *Federal programs supporting educational change.* Santa Monica, CA: Rand Corp.

Bloemen, P. (Ed.) (1999). *Evaluation of the TeleTOP Project, 1998-1999.* Internal report. Faculty of Educational Science and Technology, University of Twente, Enschede, The Netherlands.

Collis, B. (1998a). New wine and old bottles? Tele-learning, telematics, and the University of Twente. In F. Verdejo & G. Davies (Eds.), *The virtual campus: Trends for higher education and training* (pp. 3-17). London: Chapman & Hall.

Collis, B. (1998b). New didactics for university instruction: Why and how. *Computers & Education, 31*(4), 373-395.

Collis, B., & Moonen, J. (1994). Leadership for transition: Moving from the special project to systemwide integration with computers in education. In G. Kearsley & W. Lynch (Eds.), *Educational technology: Leadership perspectives* (pp. 113-136). Englewood Cliffs, NJ: Educational Technology Press.

Collis, B., & Van der Wende, M. (Eds.) (1999). *The use of information and communication technology in higher education: An international orientation on trends and issues.* Enschede: Centre for Research in Higher Education. Retrieved August 30, 2000, from the World Wide Web: *http://education2.edte.utwente.nl/ictho.nsf/framesform*

De Boer, W. F., & Collis, B. (1999). Scaling up from the pioneers: The TeleTOP method at the University of Twente. *Interactive Learning Environments, 7*(2-3), 93-112.

De Boer, W. F., & Collis, B. (2000, June). *The adaptation and use of a WWW-based course management system within two different types of faculties at the University of Twente.* Paper presented at ED-MEDIA 2000, Montreal.

Fisser, P., Van de Kamp, I., & Slot, C. (1999). *Evaluation of TeleTOP at the Faculty of Telematics.* Internal report. Enschede, NL: DINKEL Institute, University of Twente.

Fullan, M. (1991). *The meaning of educational change.* New York: Teachers College Press.

House, E. R. (1974). *The politics of educational innovation.* Los Angeles, CA: McCutchan Publications.

Messing, J., & Collis, B. (2000). *Usage, attitudes, and workload implications for a Web-based learning environment.* Paper submitted for publication. Faculty of Educational Science and Technology, University of Twente, Enschede, NL.

Plomp, T. (1992). *Ontwerpen van onderwijs en training [Design of education and training].* Utrecht, NL: Lemma.

Rosenblum, S., & Louis, K. S. (1981). *Stability and change: Innovation in an educational context.* New York: Plenum Press.

Tielemans, G., & Collis, B. (1999). Strategic requirements for a system to generate and support WWW-based environments for a faculty. In B. Collis & R. Oliver (Eds.), *Proceedings of Ed-Media '99 Seattle, World Conference on Educational Multimedia* (pp. 346-351). Charlottesville, VA: AACE. ISBN 1-880094-35-5.

Van der Veen, J., & De Boer, W. F. (1999). *Final report of the project World Wide WWW Learning Support (W3LS)*. Enschede, NL: University of Twente Educational Centre.

Visscher, A. (1999). The implications of how school staff handle information for the usage of school information systems. *International Journal of Educational Research, 25*(4), 323-334.

Chris Hughes
Lindsay Hewson

Structuring Communications to Facilitate Effective Teaching and Learning Online

SUMMARY. The current shift to mediated and WWW-based teaching and learning requires both teachers and learners to adapt established classroom practice to the new online environment. Many of the electronic systems currently on offer fail to support the complexity of interaction necessary to facilitate deep learning. This paper identifies the instructional strategies or "micro-genres" that form the essence of successful classroom teaching, and describes an online system, WebTeach™, that attempts to provide structured teacher-learner interactions that build on the familiar activities and strategies of the classroom. Through access to these "micro-genres" in an online classroom, both teacher and learner can reduce the cognitive demands of learning new processes while focusing on strategies for deep learning related to the content of the course. *[Article copies available for a fee from The Haworth Document Delivery Service: 1-800-342-9678. E-mail address: <getinfo@haworthpressinc.com> Website: <http://www.HaworthPress.com> © 2001 by The Haworth Press, Inc. All rights reserved.]*

KEYWORDS. Online, learning, structured interaction, software, Internet

CHRIS HUGHES is Senior Lecturer, Faculty of Medicine, University of New South Wales, Sydney 2052, Australia (E-mail: c.hughes@unsw.edu.au).
LINDSAY HEWSON is Senior Lecturer, Faculty of Commerce and Economics, University of New South Wales, Sydney 2052, Australia (E-mail: l.hewson@unsw.edu.au).

[Haworth co-indexing entry note]: "Structuring Communications to Facilitate Effective Teaching and Learning Online." Hughes, Chris, and Lindsay Hewson. Co-published simultaneously in *Computers in the Schools* (The Haworth Press, Inc.) Vol. 17, No. 3/4, 2001, pp. 147-158; and: *The Web in Higher Education: Assessing the Impact and Fulfilling the Potential* (ed: Cleborne D. Maddux, and D. LaMont Johnson) The Haworth Press, Inc., 2001, pp. 147-158. Single or multiple copies of this article are available for a fee from The Haworth Document Delivery Service [1-800-342-9678, 9:00 a.m. - 5:00 p.m. (EST). E-mail address: getinfo@haworthpressinc.com].

147

Teachers and students in the classroom employ a wide range of communicative devices to achieve effective live interaction and learning. Evident within the highest level of classroom communication (genre), there are a number of what we might call micro-genres–discrete communicative protocols, understood by both teachers and learners, that achieve a specific educational outcome. These have also been termed pedagogical techniques (Paulsen, 1999) or "approaches" (Laird, 1985), and highlight the essential role of communication in facilitating learning.

A simple example will indicate the richness and complexity of good classroom practice. A teacher decides to ask an important question of the class, hopefully one requiring some level of synthesis or analysis for a response (Bateman, 1990). The teacher stands in front of the class for such an event in order to gain everyone's attention. S/he may give some background information to set the context, and then pose a question, speaking clearly and choosing the words carefully to ensure appropriate cognitive processes are elicited as students attempt a response. In good practice, a wait time (Tobin, 1987) is implemented either by indicating verbally that no one is yet to answer, or by a gesture (perhaps by holding up an open hand, palm out). Students may ask clarifying questions that cause the teacher to suspend the constraints of the micro-genre for a moment while clarification is sought and explanations are given. Then, the constraints are reinstated. When the teacher judges that all understand and that enough time has been given to allow students to formulate an answer, he or she usually seeks responses from the group. Typically, not everyone offers a public answer, even though all may have prepared one. When answers are taken, they provide a form of feedback to all students to guide their evaluation of their own responses, whether publicly given or not. After answers are heard, the teacher may comment or solicit further responses from the group, and then the micro-genre changes, perhaps to discussion. At this point, the teacher may also change his or her physical position in the room and announce the shift of micro-genre to ensure that all students understand the new communicative constraints in place: "OK, if that is true, what are the implications?" asks the teacher, sitting down with the group.

Some of the more familiar micro-genres employed in a classroom include presentations, discussions, seminars, question and answer sessions, brainstorms, small group work, debates, etc. There are many others. Each of these micro-genres imposes constraints on who can and cannot speak, on what can be said and how it is said, on the sequence of speakers, on appropriate intonations and degrees of formality, on the physical and interpersonal groupings to be employed, and so on. Teachers and students are more or less expert in interpreting and implementing the requirements of these micro-genres after years of experience in classroom settings. If the students are not familiar with a particular micro-genre, the teacher will explain its constraints and requirements before using it. In the best classroom practice, teachers combine these micro-genres to create "mathemagenic" (Rothkopf, 1970, Laurillard, 1993) activities and sessions, which facilitate and encourage learning.

The transition to more mediated learning has raised the challenge of preserving these established teaching methods in the distributed and often impersonal environment of the WWW. Some new online learning environments have the potential to revolutionize our approach to and practice of teaching and learning. The revolutionary potential of electronically mediated teaching is apparent in the language used by its proponents. Goals such as the "transformation . . . of learner resources and environments . . . ," the " . . . re-engineering of universities and related institutions . . . ," and the creation of "virtual communities" are common currency among the innovators and early adopters (Rogers, 1995) who are building and using electronic environments for teaching and learning.

Of course, the expanded use of electronic environments has its critics, and like most revolutions, is being strongly opposed in some quarters. Noble (1998) presents several cases of active opposition in the area of online education, whose champions have already claimed early victory. With the proponents being equally determined, the issues will be in contention for a good while yet, and it is not at all certain that the revolution will be successful in the end (Jonassen, 1998), nor that its success will be good for education (Winner, 1997). If major changes are to occur and be accepted by mainstream educators, whole new sets of learning and participation skills will have to be developed by teachers and students. These new competencies will build on, but go far beyond what used to be termed "*computer literacy.*"

At the same time, changes in the approach to teaching are being promoted. Both the technical limitations and the enhanced possibilities of the electronic environments are driving these changes. Many examples of online education reproduce the traditional "transmission" model of education. For example, many of the courses listed in the World Lecture Hall (1999) support learning merely by using WWW pages as a distribution mechanism for course notes and administrative information. However, some of the new environments emphasize problem-based, self-directed, autonomous, and/or resource-based learning (Relan &

Gillani, 1997). They also place increased emphasis on learner activity and responsibility for learning, and they reduce the ongoing role of the teacher significantly by their use of prepackaged materials and interactions. While aspects of these trends are to be welcomed, one has to be concerned about how the transition will be made, and whether the changes will be appropriate to all the teaching and learning situations they address. Some of the impetus for approaches, such as resource-based learning, seems to come from the efficiency of the WWW as an information retrieval and delivery mechanism, rather than from sound educational reasoning.

The trend toward increasing student responsibility is intensified by the use of standard instructional design models that predetermine the grading, sequence, and content of the bulk of the educational activities and materials. Heavily designed learning packages leave little room for spontaneous activities, for genuine dialogue, or for richly structured communication. The teacher becomes more the content expert and instructional designer, but less the active facilitator of the learning process. While the design and production values of the materials and predetermined activities are often enhanced, communication is relatively impoverished when compared to the best of face-to-face practice.

While we may accept the revolutionary potential of online electronic environments, the scale of the changes and the enthusiasm of the "early adopters" (Rogers, 1995) increase the uneasiness of many and build barriers to their participation. One problem with the revolutionary language being used is its iconoclasm. It often eschews references to familiar frameworks and practices. This can form a barrier to participation for many in the majority (Collis, 1998; Moore, 1991). More temperate language, and reference to familiar frameworks, may ease the path to participation for many.

However, it is possible to take a more evolutionary approach to the development and use of electronic environments in teaching and learning; an approach in which the best paradigms of education are adapted and extended to take advantage of the new possibilities. This can be achieved without weakening the support for the imperative of best-practice teaching. At the same time, teachers and students can take the knowledge and skills in learning that they have honed in the best traditional settings and apply them to online teaching and learning. By reducing the magnitude of the adjustments required, and by building on familiar roles and processes, we should be able to facilitate acceptance and diffusion, rather than inhibit it.

THE MICRO-GENRES
OF GOOD CLASSROOM COMMUNICATION

In most online courses and in most commercial course support packages such as Top Class™ or Lotus LearningSpace™, communication is supported by e-mail, newsgroup, or Web-conferencing tools. E-mail, newsgroups and Web conferences handle straightforward messaging and have standard structures for displaying messages using only text emphasis (boldface, underlining or indentation). But these are extremely impoverished forms of communication when compared to face-to-face communication. The reduction of communication to text and stylistic elements is a significant constraint. To see just how great the reduction is, it is necessary to examine the form and composition of face-to-face communication.

Beyond the phonetic, linguistic and extra-linguistic levels (Schultz, 1989), speech acts occur in situations that are signaled by the physical setting (in dining rooms, lecture theatres, tutorial rooms, staff offices, etc.) and by the histories, roles, knowledge, linguistic expertise and expectations of the participants. These higher-level factors are captured by concepts such as register, tenor and genre (Swales, 1990) and they affect the choices made by communicators. Clearly, live communication is achieved by the manipulation of an amazing array of variables. Written text can only capture a small part of this richness.

The example presented in the introduction of this paper demonstrates the richness of good classroom communication, and much could be lost in the translation of such micro-genres to e-mail or a newsgroup (or even worse to a question on a plain Web page). Similar analyses can be readily developed for many of the other micro-genres of classroom communication, each displaying considerable complexity and subtlety.

Some of the common micro-genres include: presentations, discussions, brainstorms, informal debates, case studies, formal debates, task setting, notices, class quizzes and informal discussion.

This is not an exhaustive list of the micro-genres employed in the best of classroom practice, but it is a good representative sample. While it would be possible to reduce all of them to explicit text and instructions so they could be implemented by standard messaging systems (see Paulsen, 1999 for some inspirational attempts by teachers to do this), it should be clear that much would be lost in the translation. In addition, the cognitive burden (Sweller, 1988) on students and teachers would be significantly increased, as they make their expert knowledge of the micro-genre explicit, and interpret the attempts of others to do the same. It would be much better if each of the above micro-genres could be implemented as they are in the classroom, with a range of structural identifiers and shared expectations and constraints to support them.

The standard Internet communication tools already offer a certain amount of structuring. Newsgroup tools structure messages into two views: message views and threaded lists. As noted above, sometimes these message views permit the inclusion of stylistic devices to enhance communication. The list views employ indenting and live linking to indicate intentional relationships between messages and to facilitate the display of the messages. For these systems to work, all messages have to be given a topic, and few systems allow for anonymous contributions.

There are, however, many more elements that can be employed to structure communication in online education. Among the elements available for deployment are the following:

1. stylistic elements including character styling and page layout, tables and indentation
2. color
3. graphic elements
4. identity and anonymity
5. conditional concealment and revelation of information
6. timing, including time frames for synchronization and sequencing of activities
7. access privileges

These elements can be deployed, just as the constitutive elements of live speech, to enrich communication and enhance its educational effectiveness.

One implementation of a range of micro-genres is described below. The processes described are taken from a working prototype called WebTeach™, developed by the authors for use in university teaching at the University of New South Wales in Australia. WebTeach™ is a WWW-based conferencing system designed specifically for educational use. It is integrated with e-mail so that all contributions to the system trigger a notification message to either the whole group or to the teachers, as appropriate. All the micro-genres listed previously are supported by the WebTeach™ prototype as communicative templates (Hughes & Hewson, 1998). Following is a description of the key features of the latest implementation. (See Figure 1.)

FIGURE 1

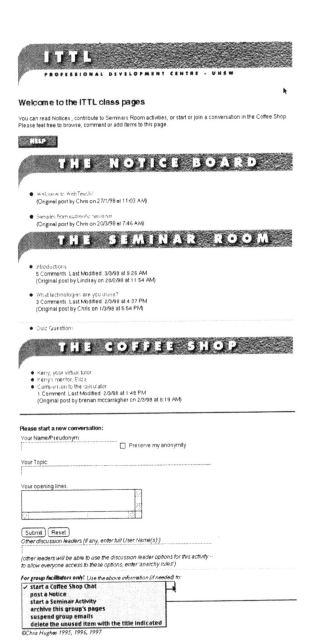

STRUCTURAL FEATURES USED
IN THE WEBTEACH™ PROTOTYPE

On entering the main group page, the student (and the teacher) is presented with a page divided into five sections. At the top is a header containing a welcome message, course logos, and links to help files and other class materials. At the bottom is a contribution form that students and teachers use to contribute new items to the page. The middle three sections comprise a virtual notice board, a virtual seminar room, and a virtual coffee shop. These areas are delineated by graphic elements.

Access to the middle areas is regulated by role. Only teachers can post notices and start seminar room activities; whereas, all participants can start coffee shop activities. However, teachers can nominate students as leaders for seminar room activities, and anyone can do the same for others when he or she initiates coffee shop activities. Such nominees are accorded "group leader" privileges for the activity. Thus the notice board and seminar room are reserved for formal class activities, while the coffee shop is an informal gathering place for all participants.

All items posted to the main page, whether notices, seminars, or coffee shop activities, appear as links to separate pages, just as in a newsgroup. The pedagogical techniques or micro-genres are supported within these separate pages (i.e., within the seminar room and coffee shop activities).

Each seminar room activity consists of a page containing an initial activity starter (a discussion point, some background to a case study or debate, etc.) together with a final form soliciting contributions appropriate to the micro-genre in use at the time. A menu to allow micro-genre shifts is included in this final form for teacher or nominated student leader use. Seminar activities may be started as discussions, case studies, or debates. Thereafter, all micro-genres are available in all activities. The same arrangement applies to coffee shop activities–they support all the micro-genres available in seminar room activities, with the teacher functions being allocated to whomever initiated the activity, and to their nominees. This allows students to use the full range of micro-genres in their own activities. However, in the following, the focus will be on the use of the micro-genres in the seminar room.

The WebTeach™ system includes a range of basic functions (not directly accessible by users) which are combined into standard structures in support of the micro-genres. These functions include the ability to:

1. display contributions as text, as table items, and as ordered or un-ordered list items
2. suppress the identity of the contributor, either automatically or on request
3. withhold contributions until their display is requested by any of those holding teacher privileges for the activity
4. employ character styles when displaying a contribution, including bold face, italics and color
5. convert embedded URLs to links and images, and e-mail addresses to "mailto:" tags
6. withhold access to a page until a contribution has been received
7. preface contributions with automatically generated text
8. sequence activities automatically
9. generate e-mail messages addressed to either the whole group, or to those nominated as teachers for the group, notifying contributions.

These functional abilities are combined to generate support for a wide range of micro-genres. Some examples are described below.

Discussion

Contributions to a discussion are displayed as unordered list items, with the identity of the contributor displayed unless anonymity is requested. Meta-comments, which address the learning process rather than the content of the discussion, are displayed in blue text as unordered list items at a second level of indentation. Contributions trigger a notification to the whole group by e-mail.

Brainstorms

A bold-typeface statement signals that the teacher has initiated a brainstorm on a topic. Attention is gained by an e-mail notification. Contributions are explicitly solicited as "ideas" and are displayed in table form below the trigger material. Identity is automatically suppressed. Meta-comments are displayed in blue as unordered list items at a second level of indentation and the table is broken for this purpose.

Formal Questions

A bold-typeface statement signals that the teacher has asked a formal question. Attention is gained by an e-mail notification. Responses are not displayed upon receipt but are stored on the server and an e-mail notification is sent to the teacher. Teachers and their nominees can view the stored responses at any time. When the teacher submits an instruction to end the "wait time" the responses are displayed in table form, with identifiers, and an e-mail notification is dispatched to the group. During the wait time, all meta-comments contributed are displayed as for the other micro-genres.

Informal Debates

A bold-faced statement preceding the trigger text signals the initiation of this micro-genre, and arguments for or against the proposition are required by the final form. Attention is gained by an e-mail notification. Contributors must indicate whether they are arguing for or against the proposition (or the contribution will be rejected), and contributions are displayed in unordered list format, preceded by a statement indicating the chosen side. Normal e-mail notifications are made for all contributions.

Formal Debates

The initial proposition is displayed as straight text, full width, and the final form seeks the initial case for the affirmative. Attention is again gained by e-mail notifications. Cases submitted are displayed in a table format with identifiers, preceded by a bold-faced statement indicating from which side the case was submitted. Meta-comments break the table format and are displayed as before. The system automatically seeks alternate cases for and against the proposition, and final summaries. After the final summaries are received and displayed, the system automatically switches the micro-genre to discussion.

Quiz Items

Within the seminar room, WebTeach™ supports a quiz facility for short-answer questions. Teachers may submit items, together with suggested responses. Only the item is displayed to students on a separate page, and responses are sought. Once a student has submitted a response, he or she can view the suggested response (or criteria) together with all other responses submitted (without author identification). This allows for formative feedback to students on their own and their peers' work. Responses are displayed in ordered list format. Teachers can view all responses, with author identification, at any time for assessment purposes. The quiz facility also supports a separate area for student quiz items. Students can use this area for developing revision questions for use by their peers. Responses to quiz items trigger e-mail notifications to the class teacher(s) only.

The WebTeach™ system supports other micro-genres, including task setting and case studies. The list is being added to as teachers identify needs. No essentiality is claimed for the structural and stylistic elements used to support and signal the micro-genres; clearly these deployments could be altered.

The system is in use by teachers in a range of schools and faculties of the University of New South Wales, including Philosophy, Psychiatry, French, Education, Food Technology and Business Studies. Teachers and students report considerable satisfaction with the system. None of the teachers are especially computer literate, but all have made the transition to online teaching with relative ease, and with little support beyond a help page. A demonstration version of the system is available at *http://www.online.unsw.edu.au/webteachdemo/welcome.html*.

By building on and extending the best of classroom teaching practice, the WebTeach™ system is intended to scaffold (Ausubel, 1960; Brown, Collins, & Duguid, 1989) support for teachers and students as they tackle the challenges of online education. Not only do the WWW-based micro-genres hold out the hope of increasing the pedagogical effectiveness of educational communication online, they also ease the transition to this mode for teachers in the early and late majority.

REFERENCES

Ausubel, D. P. (1960). The use of advance organizers in the learning and retention of meaningful verbal material. *Journal of Educational Psychology, 51*(5), 267-272.

Bateman, W. L. (1990). *Open to question: The art of teaching and learning by inquiry.* San Francisco: Jossey-Bass.

Brown, J. S., Collins, A., & Duguid, P. (1989). Situated cognition and the culture of learning. *Educational Researcher, 18*(1), 32-42.

Collis, B. (1998). Implementing change throughout the faculty: Combining educational principles, strategy and technology. In R. M. Cordery (Ed.), *The 15th Annual Conference of the Australasian Society for Computers in Learning in Tertiary Education (ASCILITE '98)* (pp. 15-22). Wollongong, Australia: University of Wollongong.

Ferguson, N. (1972). *Teaching English as a foreign language: Theory and practice.* Lausanne, Switzerland: Foma.

Hughes, C., & Hewson, L. (1998). Online interactions: Developing a neglected aspect of the virtual classroom. *Educational Technology, 38*(4), 48-55.

Jonassen, D. H. (1998). The future of technology in education: A post-modern problem with a transformative solution or whoever controls the technology creates the reality. In R. M. Cordery (Ed.), *The 15th Annual Conference of the Australasian Society for Computers in Learning in Tertiary Education (ASCILITE '98)* (pp. 29-36). Wollongong, Australia: University of Wollongong.

Laird, D. (1985). *Approaches to training and development.* Reading, MA: Addison-Wesley.

Laurillard, D. (1993). *Rethinking university teaching: A framework for the effective use of educational technology.* London: Routledge.

Moore, G. A. (1991). *Crossing the chasm.* New York: Harper Business.

Noble, D. F. (1998). *Digital diploma mills, Part III: The bloom is off the rose* [Online]. Available: *http://www.lmu.ac.uk/natfhe/nddm.htm*

Paulsen, M. F. (1999). The online report on pedagogical techniques for computer-mediated communication. [Online]. Available: *http://home.nettskolen.nki.no/~morten/*

Ramsden, P. (1992). *Learning to teach in higher education.* London: Routledge.

Relan, A., & Gillani, B. B. (1997). Web-based instruction and the traditional classroom: Similarities and differences. In B. K. Khan (Ed.), *Web-based instruction* (pp. 41-58). Englewood Cliffs, NJ: Educational Technology Publications.

Rogers, E. M. (1995). *The diffusion of innovation* (4th ed.). New York: The Free Press.

Rothkopf, E. (1970). The concept of mathemagenic activities. *Review of Educational Research, 40*(3), 325-335.

Schultz, B. G. (1989). *Communicating in the small group: Theory and practice.* New York, NY: Harper Collins.

Swales, J. M. (1990). *Genre analysis: English in academic and research settings.* Cambridge, MA: Cambridge University Press.

Sweller, J. (1988). Cognitive load during problem solving: Effects on learning. *Cognitive Science, 12,* 32-40.

Tobin, K. (1987). The role of wait time in higher cognitive learning. *Review of Educational Research, 57*(1), 69-95.

Winner, L. (1997). The handwriting on the wall: Resisting technoglobalism's assault on education. In M. Moll (Ed.), *Tech high: Globalization and the future of Canadian education* (pp. 167-188). Ottawa: Fernwood Publications.

World Lecture Hall (1999). University of Texas [Online]. Available: *http://www.utexas.edu/world/lecture/*

Susan Colaric
David Jonassen

Information Equals Knowledge, Searching Equals Learning, and Hyperlinking Is Good Instruction: Myths About Learning from the World Wide Web

SUMMARY. In this paper, we claim that too much Web-based instruction assumes that the World Wide Web is a vast library that can be used to convey knowledge, that searching and finding information on the Web equals learning, and that hyperlinking is good instruction. Based on constructivist assumptions, we critique these assumptions and offer instructional methods to counteract their effects. *[Article copies available for a fee from The Haworth Document Delivery Service: 1-800-342-9678. E-mail address: <getinfo@haworthpressinc.com> Website: <http://www.HaworthPress.com> © 2001 by The Haworth Press, Inc. All rights reserved.]*

KEYWORDS. Information searching, meaning making, constructivism, self-reflective learning, World Wide Web

SUSAN COLARIC is Doctoral Candidate, Instructional Systems Department, College of Education, 315 Keller Bldg., Penn State University, University Park, PA 16802 (E-mail: scolaric@psu.edu).
DAVID JONASSEN is Distinguished Professor, School of Information Science and Learning Technologies, University of Missouri-Columbia, 111 London Hall, Columbia, MO 65211 (E-mail: Jonassen@missouri.edu).

[Haworth co-indexing entry note]: "Information Equals Knowledge, Searching Equals Learning, and Hyperlinking Is Good Instruction: Myths About Learning from the World Wide Web." Colaric, Susan, and David Jonassen. Co-published simultaneously in *Computers in the Schools* (The Haworth Press, Inc.) Vol. 17, No. 3/4, 2001, pp. 159-169; and: *The Web in Higher Education: Assessing the Impact and Fulfilling the Potential* (ed: Cleborne D. Maddux, and D. LaMont Johnson) The Haworth Press, Inc., 2001, pp. 159-169. Single or multiple copies of this article are available for a fee from The Haworth Document Delivery Service [1-800-342-9678, 9:00 a.m. - 5:00 p.m. (EST). E-mail address: getinfo@haworthpressinc.com].

159

Learning through the Internet via the World Wide Web (Web) has expanded phenomenally in recent years. This phenomenon is found in K-12 schools and especially post-secondary institutions. The belief is that the Internet, a complex network of independent computers, can transform learning and educational opportunities for students of all ages.

Since 1994 the federal government has pursued the goal of connecting every public K-12 school to the Internet. The rationale is to broaden the resources available to teachers and students in an effort to increase students' knowledge base and prepare them for a more technological workplace (U.S. Department of Education, 1999a). By the fall of 1998, 89% of public schools were connected (U.S. Department of Education, 1999b).

Colleges and universities have preceded public schools in connectivity and are now offering instruction via the Web. In 1995 the National Center for Education Statistics conducted a Survey on Distance Education Courses Offered by Higher Education Institutions, using the Postsecondary Education Quick Information System (PEQIS). At that time, a third of the institutions in the database offered online courses, with 14% of those offering the instruction via two-way online interactions. Seventy-one percent of these institutions planned to start or increase the number of courses offered in this manner over the next three years (U.S. Department of Education, 1998). Early in the 21st century, an overwhelming majority of universities offer some form of online instruction, with many major universities offering numerous degree programs online. Our experience with designing for and teaching in four of those programs indicates that the primary method of course and program development is to convert lecture materials to Web presentation, linking course Web sites to related Web sites, constructing online examinations of knowledge acquisition, and providing some form of conferencing system to enable student questions or feedback. In developing these courses and programs, the implied goal is to replicate the classroom experience.

Underlying the phenomenal growth of online courses and Web-based instructional development are three tacit assumptions and beliefs that the online educators make when providing instruction on the Web:

1. that the World Wide Web is a vast library that can be used to convey knowledge,
2. that searching and finding information on the Web equals learning, and
3. that hyperlinking is good instruction.

We contend that these beliefs are really myths about learning that also underlie face-to-face instruction; that no theoretical or empirical research supports them; that they perpetuate the worst aspects of traditional, face-to-face education, and that the persistence of these myths will only retard the opportunities that exist when the Web is used effectively.

In the remainder of this paper, we briefly describe each myth and provide methods for counteracting its effects.

MYTH 1: THE WEB IS A VAST LIBRARY THAT CAN BE USED TO CONVEY KNOWLEDGE

Teachers and professors universally provide assignments that require their students to log on to the Web and search for information in order to write papers, solve problems or gain knowledge. Such assignments contain two fallacies: that the information on the Web is comparable to that found in libraries, and that information is the same as knowledge. The first part of this myth, that the Web is similar to a library, is false. When viewed from an educational perspective, the landscape of publicly available sites on the World Wide Web contains more landfills than libraries.

Traditionally, libraries acquired the resources on their shelves through publishers who were obliged to review and edit books in order to ensure their accuracy and reliability. The librarian then offered a second "review" of the material before it was purchased and made available in the library. Librarians also frequently review the items currently available and purge outdated, discredited, or damaged materials. This process is the antithesis of the Web. The freedom to publish information on the Web is unlimited, and there is no oversight. People have been known to publish professional-looking sites that contain biased information, incorrect or incomplete data, pranks, contradictions, out-of-date information, unauthorized revisions, and factual errors (Fitzgerald, 1997; Oppenheimer, 1997). Also, once a site is "posted," it rarely comes down, even when outdated. In order to find reliable information each Web site needs to be examined with a critical eye–a much more critical eye than most people are accustomed to using when viewing library sources.

The second part of this myth is that accessing many Web sites necessarily results in learning. However, philosophically, psychologically, and practically, information does not equal knowledge. Information, as found on any Web site, reflects what *someone else* knows and conveys (however poorly or expertly); knowledge is something that is constructed by an individual based on personal and socially mediated interpretations of experiences. This belief about meaning making is based on the constructivist assumptions that reality (the sense that we make of the world) is in the mind of the knower, so, knowledge cannot be transmitted (Jonassen, 1991). This belief system has become increasingly popular in schools and universities. In the entire history of learning research, there is no evidence that telling someone something (whether face-to-face or online) results in understanding equivalent to the teller's. When helping students to learn, teachers need to initiate the knowledge construction process by helping students to discover the dissonance between what they know and what they observe or question in their environment, and, by clarifying the dissonance between what they know and what they need to know. So a learner, carefully viewing a Web site, observes what is stated; compares the information to his or her own personal knowledge base; and, if there is dissonance, begins the process of learning and constructing new knowledge. Real meaning making (resolving the dissonance between what we know for sure and what we perceive or what we believe that others know) results from a puzzlement (Duffy & Cunningham, 1996), a perturbation (Maturana, 1983), expectation violations (Schank, 1986), adaptation to the environment which engages cycles of assimilation and accommodation (Piaget, 1985). Learners can memorize ideas that others tell them, but making meaning about phenomena involves some reflection and reconciliation of learning needs, information found, and interpretations of each. Dissonance between what is known and what is needed allows the learner to assimilate the new information, consider the various dimensions presented, and construct new meaning (knowledge) that she or he now owns. So the viewing of information on a Web site can only be used in meaningful learning if the learner is motivated to activate previous knowledge and to evaluate and transform information into knowledge–not just find the right answer to fulfill a professor's assignment.

Counteracting the Myth

Understanding the structure and nature of the World Wide Web is the first step in dispelling the myth about the Web being a library. Once students understand that there is no "authority" approving the information on the Web, they are likely to increase their cynicism for the information they find. Students must become critical theorists when using the

Web. One way to do this would be to have the students construct and publish their own Web sites. This way, they can see first-hand the unregulated nature of the Web and they may lower their expectations of the quality of its resources (Jacobson & Ignacio, 1997).

An antidote to equating information with learning is to require students to articulate the differences between what they know and what they need to know–that is, requiring learners to articulate an intention for seeking information in the first place. Until (a) students articulate what they need to know about some phenomenon, (b) develop a research strategy and execute it, and (c) consciously reflect on the meaning of the information uncovered in their search, little real learning will occur. Humans are distinct from primates in their abilities to articulate an intention and then to willfully plan to act on it. So, before beginning a search, students must generate a statement of purpose. What are they trying to prove?

MYTH 2: SEARCHING EQUALS LEARNING

In order to "learn" from the Web, it is necessary to first find information on the Web. When a teacher asks students to use the Web to find an answer, the teacher most likely (a) assumes that the student is using problem-solving skills to define the problem, choose search terms, make judgments about relevancy, and (b) expects that the student will extrapolate the information from the various sites that are found. The research, however, doesn't show this. Students are searching for *that* answer and copying it down–they are not comprehending or reflecting on the meaning of what they have found. Their intention is to complete the assignment–to find the one answer that the teacher is looking for (Bilal, 1998; Fidel, Davies, Douglass, Kohlder, Hopkins, Kushner, Miyagishima, & Toney, 1999; Schacter, Chung & Dorr, 1998). This searching for the "right" answer results in fast clicking with no possibility for learning. Simply asking students to find information on the Web will probably not result in learning.

Counteracting the Myth

It is possible to dispel this myth and engage students as active learners as they search the Web by using intentional information search skills (Jonassen, 1999). As mentioned before, the key to knowledge construction is a motivation to understand a particular problem; to identify discrepancies between what is known and what needs to be known; and to find, evaluate, and transform information into knowledge as the learner develops a solution. This can be accomplished through intentional information searching by following a four-step process: (a) plan, (b) use strategies to search the Web, (c) evaluate, and (d) triangulate sources. In addition, learners must be actively engaged in reflection to continuously review the information they find as well as the progress made toward their goal.

In planning a search, students are required to identify the dissonance between what they know and what they need to know. During this stage, several problem-solving-level processes are required. These processes can be modeled by the teacher to demonstrate the thinking that is required for a successful search. In the planning phase the learner needs to articulate her or his intention and verbalize what she or he is looking for, as well as *why* that information is needed. This thought-process activates knowledge that the learner already has and clarifies for the learner the dissonance that exists. Having students articulate their thoughts to a peer has been shown to promote better information processing at this stage (Kuhlthau, 1997).

Next, the learner must develop a conscious and intentional search strategy in order to locate information sources that may be useful. Selection of search terms can be a difficult process, and the results from studies on children's selection of search terms is mixed. Gary Marchioni (1989), in researching elementary school children's use of a full-text electronic encyclopedia, found that most students were able to successfully identify key facts and select search terms, although younger searchers (nine years old) used sentences and phrases rather than individual keywords. Spavold's research with nine-to-eleven year olds working with a database of census material supported this finding (Spavold, 1990). However, Moore and St. George (1991) reported that the selection of search terms may be beyond the ability of many 10-12 year olds; although all students were able to identify what they thought was an appropriate term, more than one-third of the words the children selected were inappropriate as judged by an adult rater. This supported Moore's earlier research where the children had difficulty generating alternative terms and 70% of those generated would not access any points in the Dewey Decimal Classification System (Moore, 1988). In light of this research, the teacher may wish to model for the students the process of asking questions such as who, where, when, and what in order to identify search terms that are associated with the problem. These terms can then be developed into a search string that would be appropriate to use in a search engine.

When Web sites are located, the information contained in them must be evaluated. That evaluation process should engage the learner in two separate aspects of evaluation–relevancy and credibility. First, is the information on the site related to the problem? Does it contribute to the intention of the search? That is, does the site contain information that pertains to the learner's expressed intention? Does it provide an explanation, examples, alternative perspectives or other pieces of information that the learner can use to construct his or her own knowledge?

Second, it is necessary that learners evaluate the credibility of the information. Evaluation of credibility usually involves two processes– evaluating the source of the information and evaluating the treatment of the subject. The teacher can model for the students the process of dissecting a Web site and should provide guiding questions to help students identify what to look for. In fact, the use of guiding questions to prime students to evaluate information more closely has been shown to be effective in children as young as five (Baker, 1984). Examples of questions to evaluate the source of the information include:

1. Does the site author have authority in that field?
2. If the site is published by an organization, is it one you recognize?
3. Does the organization have a vested interest or bias concerning the information presented?
4. Is the site owner affiliated with an organization (such as an educational institution or government agency) that has authority in the stated subject area?
5. Is it clear when the site was developed and last updated?
6. Is a bibliography or resource list included?
7. Are the references used in the bibliography credible?

Examples of questions to evaluate the treatment of the subject include:

1. Is the content factual, or opinion?
2. Does it follow a logical presentation of sequence?
3. Is the intended audience clear?
4. Are there any gaps in logic or is there missing information that is relevant to the subject?
5. Are there political or ideological biases?

6. Is this primarily an advertising or marketing site?
7. Is the language used inflammatory or extreme?
8. Is the text well written? Are there misspellings or is poor grammar used?

In asking the learner to evaluate for relevancy and credibility, you are asking him or her to engage in reflective thinking about what is really needed and what is missing. You are also asking the student to question the authority of the documents and to become more information literate by critically evaluating sources of information (Healy, 1998). A final step in this process is to triangulate the search–identify other sources that support the information found (Jonassen, 1999).

MYTH 3: HYPERLINKING IS GOOD INSTRUCTION

Most instructional Web sites convey the authors' interpretations of the content being described. Their interpretation is often augmented by a list of links to other Web sites that contain information about the topic. We have witnessed numerous presentations of instructional Web sites that proudly point to a number of other informational Web sites. What is disturbing is that these authors too often convey credibility in the links that they list without critically evaluating the information contained in those Web sites. And, pointing to other sites assumes that learners will access those sites and critically analyze the information contained in them as well as evaluate the information contained in them in terms of the learners' intentions. That, too, seldom occurs.

When instruction is limited to pointing at other sources of information on the WWW, students too often lose focus. Students may veer away from their original intentions and get off-task by finding information that appears more interesting. After a few diversions, they may get lost in hyperspace. Again, unless students articulate a purpose for searching and develop a plan for it, they are less likely to make meaning from their interactions.

Counteracting the Myth

By referencing other Web sites, authors need to clearly communicate their beliefs and perspectives as authors and provide access to other conflicting or alternative points of view in other Web sites that have been critically evaluated.

Another solution (not the only one) to following hyperlinks is for learners to create them. Users everywhere have begun to help each other conquer the complexities of the Web by collaborating directly or indirectly in the navigation task by e-mailing URLs to one another or creating Web sites with pointers to other Web sites of their favorite links. They are reviewed, hand-selected lists of pointers to other Web sites. This social collaboration process is known as social navigation (Dieberger, 1997). Social navigation occurs when information users collaborate directly or indirectly in the navigational task. Direct social navigation is a form of discourse community, a group of individuals with common interests who agree to share ideas and resources. A great deal of intellectual work goes into social navigation Web pages. These pages are not only a powerful form of communication but also a clear measure of understanding—that is, they can be assessed and evaluated as a measure of learning. How comprehensive are the resources? How well organized are they? How relevant are the sites; that is, how well have they been selected?

CONCLUSION

The use of the Web for disseminating information and linking to other information sites provides no real alternatives to face-to-face instruction. It is subject to the myths that we have described in this paper. But the World Wide Web can be used effectively as a learning tool if some of the methods for counteracting those myths are employed. However, it is unlikely that the Web will ever transform learning and educational opportunities for students, as some educators have predicted. Only educators can do that. Teachers need to develop lessons that engage meaning making, promote problem solving, and require critical thinking irrespective of how information is disseminated.

In order to use the Web more effectively, we recommend that teachers and professors begin by having students articulate an information need or purpose and develop a hypothesis. Then have them develop and clearly communicate a search strategy for finding the information, perhaps using a Concept Block Diagram (see Figure 1). Students must use multiple criteria for evaluating the Web sites found, assessing their relevance to the intention and dissecting the sites for evidence of credibility. Ask the students to then triangulate their information by finding three

FIGURE 1. Using a Concept Block Diagram to Identify Search Terms

A concept block diagram can help students identify key terms and alternate terms for searching. Begin with the information or hypothesis. Then determine guiding questions that explore further the information that is needed. These questions are placed across the top of the page. Next, the students generate answers and synonyms and list them in the column underneath the question. In this example students wanted to learn what fresh water crustaceans, specifically crayfish, eat so they can plan and build a terrarium for their school.

Information need: to find out about the eating habits of fresh water crustaceans

What are they?	**Where are they?**	**What do we want to know?**
crustaceans	fresh water	eat
arthropods	streams	consume
crayfish	rivers	
crawfish	lakes	

The concept block diagram can then be used to construct a search expression by placing OR between the answers that appear together vertically and linking them together with AND for each question.

(crustaceans OR arthropods OR crayfish OR crawfish) AND (fresh water OR streams OR rivers OR lakes) AND (eat OR consume)

sources that confirm the content they would like to use. Finally, encourage your students to reflect on the meaningfulness of what they have in light of their intentions. It is through thoughtful lessons such as this that *learning* can occur with the Web.

REFERENCES

Baker, L. (1984). Children's effective use of multiple standards for evaluating their comprehension. *Journal of Educational Psychology, 76,* 588-597.

Bilal, D. (1998). *Children's search processes in using World Wide Web search engines: An exploratory study.* Paper presented at American Society for Information Science '98, Pittsburgh, PA.

Dieberger, A. (1997). Supporting social navigation on the World Wide Web. *International Journal of Human-Computer Studies, 46,* 805-825.

Duffy, T.M., & Cunningham, D.J. (1996). Constructivism: Implications for the design and delivery of instruction. In D.H. Jonassen (Ed.), *Handbook of research for educational communications and technology* (pp. 170-198). New York: Macmillan.

Fidel, R., Davies, R.K., Douglass, M.H., Kohlder, J.K., Hopkins, C.J., Kushner, E.J., Miyagishima, B.K., & Toney, C.D. (1999). A visit to the information mall: Web searching behavior of high school students. *Journal of the American Society for Information Science, 50*(1), 24-37.

Fitzgerald, M.A. (1997). Misinformation on the Internet: Applying evaluation skills to online information. *Emergency Librarian, 24*(3), 9-14.

Healy, J.M. (1998). *Failure to connect: How computers affect children's minds–for better or worse.* New York: Simon & Schuster.

Jacobsen, F.E., & Ignacio, E.N. (1997). Teaching reflection: Information seeking and evaluation in a digital library environment. *Library Trends, 45*(4), 771-802.

Jonassen, D.H. (1991). Objectivism vs. Constructivism: Do we need a new paradigm? *Educational Technology: Research and Development, 39*(3), 5-14.

Jonassen, D.H. (1999). *Computers as mindtools for schools: Engaging critical thinking* (2nd Ed.). Upper Saddle River, NJ: Merrill.

Kuhlthau, C. (1997). Learning in digital libraries: An information search process approach. *Library Trends, 45,* 708-724.

Marchioni, G. (1989). Information seeking strategies of novices using a full-text electronic encyclopedia. *Journal of the American Society of Information Science, 20,* 54-66.

Maturana, H.T., & Varela, H. (1972). *The tree of life: The biological roots of human understanding.* Boston: Shambala.

Moore, P.A. (1988). Children's information seeking: Judging books by their covers. *School Library Review, 8*(5).

Moore, P.A., & St. George, A. (1991). Children as information seekers: The cognitive demands of books and library systems. *School Library Media Quarterly, 19,* 161-168.

Oppenheimer, T. (1997). The computer delusion. *The Atlantic Monthly, 280*(1), 45-62.

Schacter, J., Chung, G.K., & Dorr, A. (1998). Children's Internet searching on complex problems: Performance and process analyses. *Journal of the American Society for Information Science, 49,* 840-850.

Schank, R.C. (1982). *Dynamic memory.* Cambridge, UK: Cambridge University Press.

Spavold, J. (1990). The child as naive user: A study of database use with young children. *International Journal of Man-Machines Studies, 32,* 603-625.

U.S. Department of Education, National Center for Educational Statistics, Postsecondary Information Quick System (1998, February). *Distance education in higher education institutions: Incidence, audiences, and plans to expand* (NCES 98-132) [Online]. Available: *http://nces.ed.gov/pubs99/1999005.df*

U.S. Department of Education, Office of Educational Research and Improvement, National Center for Educational Statistics (1999a, February). *The condition of education* (NECS 1999-005) [Online]. Available: *http://nces.ed.gov/pubs99/1999005.pdf*

U.S. Department of Education, Office of Educational Research and Improvement, National Center for Educational Statistics (1999b, February). *Internet access in public schools and classrooms: 1994-1998* (NECS 1999-017) [Online]. Available: *http://nces.ed.gov/pubsearch/pubsinfo.asp?pubid=1999017*

Christine O. Cheney
Michael M. Warner
Diann N. Laing

Developing a Web-Enhanced Televised Distance Education Course: Practices, Problems, and Potential

SUMMARY. Web enhancements to university courses offered via televised distance education can address several of the problems presented by the geographical barriers inherent in this delivery system. This article describes a Web site, The Teachers Lounge, developed for a distance education course in collaboration for special education teachers. Students at six separate locations were able to interact and collaborate around case studies presented on the Web. The article describes the conceptualization and development of the site, the students' reactions to the site, and suggestions to others interested in using similar Web applications. *[Article copies available for a fee from The Haworth Document Delivery Service: 1-800-342-9678. E-mail address: <getinfo@ haworthpressinc.com> Website: <http://www.HaworthPress.com> © 2001 by The Haworth Press, Inc. All rights reserved.]*

CHRISTINE O. CHENEY is Professor, Special Education, Department of Curriculum and Instruction, College of Education, University of Nevada, Reno, NV 89557 (E-mail: cheney@unr.edu).
MICHAEL M. WARNER is Professor, Department of Curriculum and Instruction, College of Education, University of Nevada, Reno, NV 89557 (E-mail: mmwarner@ unr.edu).
DIANN N. LAING is Media Coordinator, Teaching and Learning Technologies, University of Nevada, Reno, NV 89557 (E-mail: diannl@unr.edu).

[Haworth co-indexing entry note]: "Developing a Web-Enhanced Televised Distance Education Course: Practices. Problems, and Potential." Cheney, Christine O., Michael M. Warner, and Diann N. Laing. Co-published simultaneously in *Computers in the Schools* (The Haworth Press, Inc.) Vol. 17, No. 3/4, 2001, pp. 171-188; and: *The Web in Higher Education: Assessing the Impact and Fulfilling the Potential* (ed: Cleborne D. Maddux, and D. LaMont Johnson) The Haworth Press, Inc., 2001, pp. 171-188. Single or multiple copies of this article are available for a fee from The Haworth Document Delivery Service [1-800-342-9678, 9:00 a.m. - 5:00 p.m. (EST). E-mail address: getinfo@haworthpressinc.com].

171

KEYWORDS. Televised distance education, teacher education in special education, Web-enhanced teacher education

The field of special education is facing shortages of trained personnel, and federal projections do not see this need diminishing in the near future (Boe, Cook, Bobbitt, & Terhanian, 1998; Office of Special Education Programs, 1998). Rural school districts, in particular, find it difficult to recruit and retain teachers of students with both high and low-incidence disabilities.

In an effort to meet the needs of children with disabilities with well-qualified teachers, colleges and universities are using a variety of course delivery options to prepare pre-service teachers and to provide continuing professional development to those teachers already in the field. Televised distance education courses are commonly used to support the preparation of special education teachers who live and teach far from university campuses (Spooner, Spooner, Algozzine, & Jordan, 1998). In addition, many teacher education programs are incorporating Web-based or Web-enhanced courses in an attempt to reach nontraditional students and/or practicing teachers interested in developing skills in special education (Meyen, Lian, & Tangen, 1997). Web components of courses also are seen as methods of introducing teachers to the power and potential of the Internet as a resource for their teaching.

A further trend in teacher education literature in special education is the use of case-based teaching, similar to that used in medical and business colleges (Anderson & Baker, 1999; Elksnin, 1998). Such case studies may focus on a child with disabilities and ask prospective teachers to make decisions about the child's education. Others take the perspective of a teacher who is grappling with a decision or issue related to a student, a class of students, or an aspect of working with other professionals or parents. Case-based teaching is thought by some professionals to be an effective way of enhancing the preparation of special education and general education teachers (Elksnin, 1998).

This article describes efforts to marry the three above-mentioned methodologies of televised distance education, Web-enhanced course components, and case-based instruction in the delivery of a course in special education. This effort involved the collaboration of the three authors: the course instructor, a person knowledgeable in the use of databases, and a person with expertise in graphic design. The sections that follow describe the contribution of each person to the development of a Web site called the "Teachers Lounge." Information is also presented that describes the effectiveness of the site as assessed through student surveys prior to the introduction of the Web component, as well as summative student evaluations of the Web-based activities. The final section discusses what was learned as a result of the collaboration: ways of improving Web activities and the potential of Web-enhanced instruction in courses such as the one described.

CONCEPTUALIZATION OF THE TEACHERS LOUNGE

In the spring semester of 1999, it was determined that a course within the special education sequence would be taught via televised distance education. The course covered the topic of collaboration and consultation in special education. The course was dual-listed at the graduate and undergraduate levels; therefore, it could be taken by pre-service seniors or by practicing teachers. Although the largest group of students in this televised course was in the on-campus class, there were also students attending at five remote sites throughout the state. In past semesters, group as well as individual assignments had been required for this course. Group assignments had not posed a problem when the course had been taught in a traditional, on-campus format. However, the logistics of offering such a course via distance education meant that students attending class at Site A could only collaborate with the other students at Site A. There would be no practical or economical way for them to collaborate in any meaningful way with students in the campus-based section or with those at Site B, unless some nontraditional means of collaboration were developed.

The course instructor determined that an interactive Web site could be a promising method for allowing students to collaborate across the geographical distances covered by the course. In retrospect, there would have been many ways to accomplish this goal, including the use of an e-mail-based chat room or a listserv. However, the course instructor was interested in experimenting with enhancing the course through the use of the Internet. A major reason for this decision was that the use of a Web site could model the use of the Internet with teachers who could, in turn, look at its potential for their students.

In order to prepare for the development of the course site, the instructor examined existing professional Web sites related to special education. Many of the sites that were found could be described as "a book with a different cover." They appeared as text information with links to additional text information. Largely, these included reformatted flyers, brochures, or books. Graphics on many of the academic Web sites consisted of clip art. They added color or interest to the sites, but they were not well integrated into the actual function of the sites (in contrast to many commercial or educational sites for children). It was felt that much of the potential of the Internet for persons whose literacy is affected by disability would be in the integrated use of graphics as more than adornment for the site.

In conceptualizing the site for a course on collaboration in education, it was determined that graphics would be used in an integral way. The graphical theme of the Web site would be a "Teachers Lounge." This room is where teachers often gather and discuss students, instruction, and other issues facing education. It is where collaboration, especially informal collaboration, occurs at many schools. For the course Web site, collaboration would center on a number of case studies or vignettes related to children, and these cases could grow or change over the semester. In addition, the site might be used to post class information or exchange general views not related to particular cases.

At this point, the course instructor was faced with a dilemma. While the conceptualization of the site was taking shape, the instructor did not have the technical skills to actually develop a Web site, let alone one that would enable students to collaborate with one another. Several colleagues, however, were interested in the ideas involved in the development of the Web site. One individual had set up a number of applications using the database software, FileMaker Pro (FileMaker Inc., 1998). He was very proficient with this program and felt that it had potential for storing contributions students made and allowing easy organization and access to these contributions over time. Another colleague was a graphic designer and had developed Web sites for other university programs. She was interested in experimenting with merging graphics with a database program.

Thus began collaboration among three professionals at a university to develop a Web site to enhance a course about collaboration for special education teachers. Interested readers are encouraged to visit the site in order to understand more fully its workings and its limitations (*http://casatweb.ed.unr.edu/cgi-bin/webobjects/CI743*).

CREATING THE DATABASE
FOR THE TEACHERS LOUNGE

The database side of the Teachers Lounge was created using FileMaker Pro software (FileMaker Inc., 1998). The reasons for selecting this software included the following: (a) It is relatively easy to learn and use; (b) it can be used on either a PC or a Macintosh platform; (c) it can be connected to Web pages using the Web connection functions within FileMaker itself; and (d) entries in the database can be manipulated in a variety of ways for later analysis.

A simple database was constructed that contained the following fields:

1. Date (the date a contribution was submitted to the database)
2. Time (the time of day that a contribution was submitted)
3. Name (the name of the person making the contribution)
4. E-mail (the e-mail address of the person making the contribution)
5. Vignette (the title of the particular vignette or case study that was being addressed)
6. Subject (a title that contributors used to label their message)
7. Message (the text of the message itself)

Each time someone made a contribution, a new record was created and stored in the database.

The initial Web pages for the course were created using HomePage 3.0 (FileMaker Inc., 1998). This hypertext markup language (HTML) editor was chosen because of its ease of use and because it was designed to be used in tandem with FileMaker Pro. Specifically, HomePage allows the user to write tags in HTML code that support communication between the Web page (front end) and the database (back end). Many of the Web pages were created using a wizard or "assistant" that created pages for specific communication with the database, including pages for the following:

1. Searching the database for specific contributions or sets of contributions (e.g., by date or by vignette)
2. Adding a new record to the database (for submitting a contribution)
3. Displaying the details of a particular record (for reading a contribution)

When the initial set of pages was completed, a process took place in which the pages (in HTML format) were exported to the computer used by the graphics designer. She imported these files into a different Web page program and developed the supporting graphics. The process was then reversed. The graphics designer exported the files from her program and imported them back into HomePage. The pages were tested in

HomePage and, if necessary, sent back to the designer for further development. Very few technical problems were encountered in these exchanges.

DEVELOPING THE GRAPHICS AND USER INTERFACE FOR THE TEACHERS LOUNGE

The graphics designer approached the development of the user interface for the site by asking questions about the students' perspectives: When a user accesses the site initially, where do they come in? What do they see? How is the stage set?

After discussion around those ideas, the graphics designer envisioned creating the metaphor of the Teachers Lounge. The home page would portray a door that would lead into the lounge. However, other elements that are normally on a homepage (buttons leading to other places, a description of what the site was all about, and instructions on how to proceed) would be included in the design as a natural part of the look and feel of the site, which represented a public school.

The final design of the homepage presented a door with the words "Teachers Lounge" above it (see Figure 1).

Banners on the wall beside the door were buttons that, when clicked, opened other pages, such as the university homepage and the page for other databases within the College of Education. Posted on the door of the Teachers Lounge was a notice that invited members of the class to READ. Directions for understanding the site navigation and site logistics were given in the READ notice. Passing the cursor over the notice caused the hyperlink hand to appear. Clicking on the notice brought up a new page with site instructions. Information at the end of the READ notice gave the reader instructions for entering the Teachers Lounge (the next page). It was not necessary for the user to go to the READ notice each time. Clicking on the doorknob at any time permitted entry into the lounge.

The next page was a photograph (taken at a public school with a digital camera) with graphic enhancements of two university instructors talking at a table in a real teachers lounge (Figure 2). Pictured behind them in the lounge were a bulletin board (real) and a graphically inserted file cabinet, drawn to look as if it were part of the lounge setting. Passing the cursor over either of these two objects caused a Web "rollover" to occur where text information appeared identifying the object as

FIGURE 1. Opening Page for the Teachers Lounge Web Site

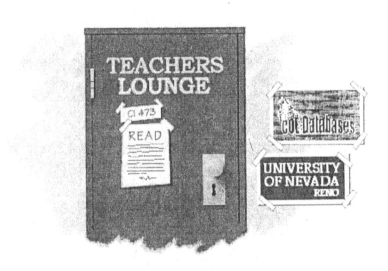

well as the traditional hyperlink hand. Clicking on either the bulletin board or the file cabinet brought up additional pages.

The bulletin board page (Figure 3) displayed items that were modified to continue the navigation opportunities: e-mail directly to the class instructor to allow for private communication; a method of posting general class notices; a path that enabled the user to move into the student vignettes; and another path that would enable the user to return to the lounge page. Clicking on the file cabinet resulted in the appearance of four file folders, each with a student's name. Clicking on a file folder tab took the user to the content information for that vignette (Figure 4). Each vignette page had a drawn graphic that portrayed the student on whom the case study focused. These drawings were done digitally using a drawing tablet.

Once on the vignette page, the end user needed to have a method of access to continue with a response, or to return to a previous point. Navigation buttons were designed graphically so that the images on each button were a visual picture of the button function: one button to move to the database side of the Web site, a bulletin board button to return to

FIGURE 2. Inside Teachers Lounge Web Site, File Cabinet, Bulletin Board, and Telephone Are Links to Other Parts of the Site

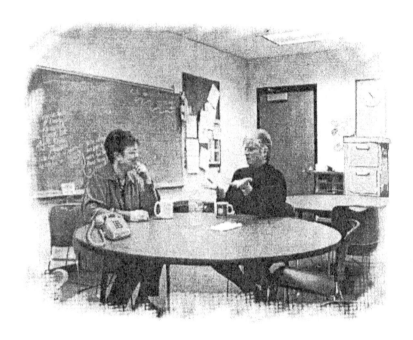

the bulletin board, a lounge picture button to return to the lounge, etc. These same return-type navigation buttons were also placed on pages developed on the database side of the site so that continuity was maintained.

The graphic development tools used with this site included the following:

1. Hardware: Macintosh G3 266mHz, 160MB RAM, 4G hard drive; CalCom 6x9 drawing tablet with cordless pen; Olympus D-600L digital camera
2. Software: Photoshop 5.0 (Adobe Systems Inc., 1998), Fractal Design Painter 5.5 (MetaCreations Corp., 1998), GoLive Cyberstudio 4.0 (Adobe Systems Inc., 1998).

FIGURE 3. Bulletin Board with Graphic Links to Other Parts of the Site

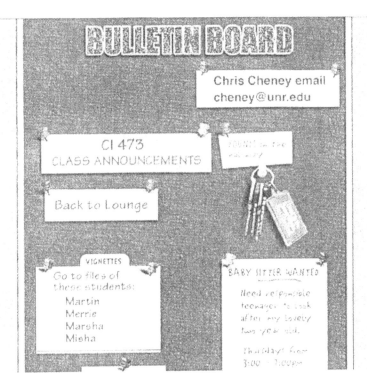

RESULTS OF THE COLLABORATION:
THE CONTENT AND USE
OF THE TEACHERS LOUNGE WEB SITE

In order to give students at all six distance-education sites focus for their collaborations, fictitious vignettes or case studies were created about four children at different grade levels: kindergarten, fourth grade, seventh grade, and eleventh grade. Two of the children were specifically identified as having disabilities, while two were described as having difficulties but here not specifically mentioned as disabled. Class participants selected one vignette to respond to over the course of the semester. The vignettes were written from the perspective of a school professional who was concerned about the student and who came to the Teachers Lounge to seek advice or information.

FIGURE 4. One of the Vignettes in the File Cabinet

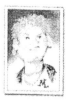

Misha

Vignette #3: Misha presents his 7th grade teachers with a real challenge

Misha Doyesky arrived at Huntley Middle School six months ago. He and his parents emigrated from Russia just over a year ago. Misha spent the first three months of the school year at an intensive English language center, but he was moved to the middle school because of his good command of the English language and his unhappiness at the center.

Misha learned to speak English in school in Russia. His skills in reading and writing are slightly better than his verbal English, but he does very well with the language. However, school rules are another story. Misha has an explosive temper. Any student who gets in his way is pushed or yelled at (in angry Russian). He rarely participates in class and pointedly looks away from teachers if they call on him. Assignments are not completed. Misha spends a lot of class time reading books in both Russian and English. Misha dresses with a "gangster" look, but he has few friends and does not seem to be affiliated with any gangs. It's easy to tell when near Misha that he smokes regularly.

Pete Groves, the Vice-Principal for discipline, has received many complaints from teachers about Misha. The teachers have been willing to give Misha time to adjust to his new environment, and they are clearly impressed with Misha's abilities with the language. However, they feel it is time that Misha begin participating in class and school activities, and his behavior is not only rude but is against school rules. Any other student displaying Misha's behavior would have been disciplined long before now.

Pete knows that something must be done about Misha. He called Misha's home, but it was clear in a minute that neither of Misha's parents speaks English. Pete wants to change Misha's behavior without "losing him." He feels Misha is a very bright but lonely student who could easily turn off to school completely. Pete walks into the Teachers' Lounge and asks if anyone would like to help him brainstorm ideas to deal with Misha.

    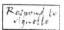

Four times during the semester, the vignettes were updated. These updates consisted of the school professional receiving a phone call from a parent, the results of testing, or of some school occurrence that led to more questions or concerns. In this manner, the students had reasons to add contributions to the Web site throughout the semester.

As part of the course requirements, students were asked to contribute to the Web site at least four times. Five points could be earned for each contribution (up to four); therefore, participation with the Web site amounted to only about 4% of the students' grade for the course.

In addition to updates and student contributions, other professionals were invited to add their perspectives to the discussions of the vignettes.

For example, the director of the university's Office of Student Support Services made comments related to the case of the eleventh-grade student with multiple disabilities who wished to go to college. A professor of literacy studies commented on the instructional approaches that might be taken with a fourth-grade student with specific learning disabilities. All contributions to the site were made by course participants and other professionals using their real names.

One unplanned event that added significantly to the relevance and saliency of the course was the use of the Web site for extended discussion of the tragedy of Columbine High School. Immediately after the shootings at Columbine High, a class discussion focused on this complex issue. As rich as this discussion was, many students had reactions or thoughts they did not share during the televised distance-education class session. At the end of the discussion, I mentioned that we could continue to discuss this event on the Web site. A large number of students chose to do so. One student even raised the issue of peer acceptance and ostracism among the students within the college. This generated quite a bit of discussion and reflection on personal behavior.

STUDENT REACTIONS
TO THE TEACHERS LOUNGE WEB SITE

A total of 56 students were enrolled in the course at all six sites. The demographics of the students are presented in Table 1.

Students were asked to complete a brief survey about their use of the Internet prior to the launching of the Web site. Fifty-three students (95%) completed the anonymous survey. Table 2 presents a summary of the survey results.

Students were evenly divided on whether they would be accessing the Web site at home, at school (computer lab or library), or at both places. It was more common for the on-campus students (who were largely undergraduates) to use their personal computers, rather than those at a school, lab, or library. Practicing teachers were apt to use their classroom computers, if these computers were connected to the Internet. The majority of students reported using online services daily or several times per week for e-mail, research, and/or services such as banking or travel. Most students had never taken a course that had an Internet or Web site component. However, the vast majority of students reported little or no anxiety about the Internet component of this course,

TABLE 1. Demographics of the Students Enrolled in the Collaboration Course Using the Teachers Lounge Web Site

	On-campus	Site A	Site B	Site C	Site D	Site E	Total
Distance from campus		80 mi.	165 mi.	130 mi.	30 mi.	60 mi.	
Students Enrolled	27	9	5	3	9	3	56
Pre-service teachers	24	0	0	1	3	2	30
Practicing teachers	3	9	5	2	6	1	26

although three students stated they had very high levels of anxiety about using the Web site.

At the end of the semester, students were asked to anonymously evaluate the Web site component of the course through a questionnaire. A total of 91% of the students completed this evaluation. Several major themes emerged, defined as similar comments mentioned by three or more students. These results are presented in Table 3. The evaluation was divided into questions about the vignettes, the bulletin board, and changes in the students' level of comfort or anxiety about using an interactive Web site.

The questions about the vignettes revealed that approximately equal numbers of students responded to each of the four vignettes. One student chose to respond to all four vignettes and one student reported reading but not responding to any of the vignettes. The students also were asked to comment on the most interesting or effective aspects of the vignettes, the least interesting or effective aspects of the vignettes, and their suggestions for improvement of the vignette activities. Several positive and negative themes emerged from these questions.

On the positive side, students enjoyed seeing others' perspectives on the situations and comparing them with their own. Students commented about the interest, realism, and quality of the vignettes. Additionally students enjoyed the comments made by professionals from outside the class and recommended adding more of these.

On the negative side, students wanted more information to react to through more frequent updates of information or having more vignettes to respond to. On a related note, they also disliked having to read all of the other students' comments (due to the large number of students enrolled in the course and the small number of vignettes). Additionally, comments were made about difficulties in accessing the site at various times over the semester.

TABLE 2. Results of the Student Survey Completed Prior to Using the Teachers Lounge Web Site

	On-campus	Site A	Site B	Site C	Site D	Site E	Totals
Percent (%) of surveys returned	92.6	100	100	100	100	66.7	94.6
Location of computer							
• Home only	14	0	0	0	5	0	19
• School/lab/library only	8	5	1	2	2	1	19
• Both places	3	4	4	1	2	1	15
Frequency of online activities							
• Daily or more	6	4	4	1	2	2	19
• Several times a week	9	2	1	1	6	0	19
• Weekly	2	0	0	0	0	0	2
• Several times a month	0	2	0	1	0	0	3
• Monthly	0	0	0	0	0	0	0
• Rarely or never	8	1	0	0	1	0	10
Types of online activities							
• Internet only	9	5	2	1	1	0	18
• E-mail only	0	0	0	1	2	0	3
• Internet, e-mail, and services	8	2	2	1	2	0	15
• Use unspecified	6	2	1	0	2	2	13
• Do not use	2	0	0	0	2	0	4
Previous courses with Internet components							
• No	17	8	5	2	7	1	40
• Yes	5	1	0	1	1	1	9
• E-mail use only	3	0	0	0	1	0	4
Anxiety level about Web site use							
• Very high	2	0	1	0	0	0	3
• Moderate	2	2	0	1	3	0	8
• Little	8	5	2	2	5	2	24
• None	13	2	2	0	1	0	18
Types of concerns							
• Equipment issues	1	1	1	0	2	0	5
• Time/forgetting	2	0	0	0	0	0	2
• Personal concerns	3	2	0	2	3	0	10
• None	19	6	4	1	4	2	36

TABLE 3. Themes that Emerged in the Student Evaluations of the Teachers Lounge Web Site

	On-Campus	Site A	Site B	Site C	Site D	Site E	Total
Percent (%) of evaluations returned	85.2	88.9	100.0	100.0	100.0	100.0	91.1
Numbers selecting each vignette							
• Kindergarten	9	2	1	0	1	3	16
• Fourth grade	7	1	2	1	1	0	12
• Seventh grade	3	1	2	0	4	0	10
• Eleventh grade	3	4	0	1	3	0	11
• None or all	1	0	0	1	0	0	2
Positive aspects of vignettes							
• Variety of viewpoints	13	3	4	2	3	2	27
• Realism/interest	6	2	2	2	4	0	16
• Responses of outside professionals	3	0	1	1	0	1	6
Negative aspects of vignettes							
• Getting through all responses	9	0	2	0	1	0	12
• Access problems	5	1	0	0	3	0	9
• More information was needed	0	2	2	0	0	0	4
Suggestions to improve							
• More up-dates or more vignettes	8	2	0	0	2	2	14
• Too many opinions given in responses	2	1	0	0	1	0	4
Frequency of Bulletin Board use							
• Never	4	2	0	0	1	0	7
• 1-3 times total	5	2	1	1	2	1	12
• Regularly (not specific)	4	4	0	1	5	2	16
• Each time logged on	10	0	0	1	1	0	12
Level of comfort about use of Web site							
• No change	5	4	0	1	2	0	12
• More comfort	18	3	5	2	6	3	37
• High anxiety	0	0	0	0	1	0	1

Questions about the bulletin board component of the Web site indicated that these class announcements were not accessed as often as the vignettes. Almost 40% of the students reported that they either never checked the announcements or checked them three times or less during the semester. Eleven specific suggestions were made for improving the bulletin board; however, only two of them, posting reminders about assignments that were due and announcing events related to special education that were occurring throughout the area, were suggested by more than one person.

Thirty-seven students indicated that the activities increased their comfort about using an interactive Web site or made general positive comments about the site. Twelve students reported that the assignment did not change their level of comfort, while one student indicated that this was a very difficult and uncomfortable activity.

SUGGESTIONS FOR IMPROVING
WEB-BASED COURSE COMPONENTS

Web-based course components have great potential to enhance distance education courses in special education. Based on experiences with this course, suggestions for others who may be interested in developing similar course activities fall into four areas: (a) the importance of professional collaboration in developing Web activities, (b) the creation and maintenance of the cases (vignettes), (c) the logistics of how students access and use the site, and (d) dreams about future uses of the Teachers Lounge Web site.

The Importance of Collaboration

The creation of the Teachers Lounge Web site was a collaborative effort, and it would not exist without the work of all three people involved. As colleges and universities make more use of the Internet for the complete or partial delivery of courses, instructors should have access to other professionals with supporting skills. If Web-based course components are to have flexible applications for both course content and analysis of student responses, persons with expertise in various software applications are needed. If these course components are to involve more than text and use graphics in a unified and integral manner, persons with design expertise also should be involved.

Professionals in all fields are becoming more adept with the application of computer technology. However, the most effective and rewarding components of the development of this Web site came as a result of the collaboration, brainstorming and speculating that was done as a team. The authors were able to accomplish more work of higher quality by using one another's skills. In addition, all learned more about hardware, software, and Web sites than we could have by working alone.

Creation and Maintenance of Case Studies

Case studies seem to be an effective focus for Web-based interactions of students in a course such as the one described. However, it is vital that the cases or vignettes created for the Web site be interesting, realistic, and dynamic. We found that drawings of the fictitious students were appreciated, but other elements such as student records, test results, and Individual Educational Plans would have enhanced the cases. Two of the practicing teachers enrolled in the class reported that collaborating on a fictitious case was not helpful to them when they were faced daily with real students. Others, however, reported that the cases helped them make applications to their own students.

In retrospect it is clear that four cases were not enough for a class of over 50 students. While this number of cases ensured that students from various sites had to collaborate with each other, it lead to too many responses for students to read–especially if they had not visited the site for a week or more. It also became clear that the cases had to be updated more frequently than four times during the semester. Having professionals from outside the class respond to the vignettes added new information to the sites and new perspectives that many students enjoyed.

The Logistics of Student Use of the Site

One of the shortcomings of the Web site was that some students had difficulty accessing the site, especially early in the semester. This was partially due to the refinements we made in the site (taking the site offline while these were completed) and partially due to some equipment incompatibilities with the computers in the library at one of the remote sites.

Students were asked to respond to the vignettes at least four times during the semester, but no other parameters were put on this requirement. As a result, some students reported that they often forgot to check the site regularly. About six students (all pre-service teachers) made all four of their responses within the last two weeks of the semester, obviously not appreciating the collaborative emphasis of the activity. In the future, additional guidance will be given to the students, including more discussion of the site and written suggestions/guidelines for the students' responses. These suggestions will include asking the students to do the following: space their responses out over the entire semester, apply specific techniques and information learned in class to the cases, carefully reflect on what others have said before responding, and research specific information about aspects of the cases (as opposed to merely listing what needs to be found, posing questions, or stating opinions).

Future Applications of the Teachers Lounge Web Site

The original goal for the Web site was for it to negate the barrier of distance among the members of the class. As the site was used, however, it became evident that it could transcend other barriers as well. The most obvious extension of the site is to use it for collaboration among the members of more than one class, in more than one academic discipline. Currently, plans are underway for graduate students in a course in school counseling to also contribute to the site. It is not much of a stretch to include students in a variety of related fields such as general education, school psychology, educational administration, speech pathology, etc. In this manner, professionals of varying perspectives are involved in collaborations centered on students with special needs.

Because location is not a limiting factor in the use of a Web site, students from other universities or regions of the country could also be involved. This would enable students to hear voices that reflect diversity not represented in a local community. Former students or practicing teachers who are not enrolled in the course could contribute to the case studies or be asked to relate the vignettes to situations in their own schools. The authors of the course texts, nationally known authorities in relevant subjects, and policymakers can all be invited to contribute to discussions on a course Web site.

In conclusion, as university instructors experiment with this powerful new technology, many will need considerable support to be able to realize their visions. Not everyone has or needs expertise in developing high-quality Web-enhanced courses. Giving university faculty access to others who have this expertise is essential, however, if educators are to get the most out of this exciting and dynamic technology.

REFERENCES

Anderson, P.L., & Baker, B.K. (1999). A case-based curriculum approach to special education teacher preparation. *Teacher Education and Special Education, 22,* 188-192.

Boe, E.E., Cook, L.H., Bobbitt, S.A., & Terhanian, G. (1998). The shortage of fully certified teachers in special education. *Teacher Education and Special Education, 21,* 1-21.

Elksnin, L.K. (1998). Use of the case method of instruction in special education teacher preparation programs: A preliminary investigation. *Teacher Education and Special Education, 21,* 95-108.

FileMaker Pro 4.0 [Computer software]. (1998). Santa Clara, CA: FileMaker, Inc.

Fractal Design Painter 5.5.012. [Computer software]. (1998). Carpinteria, CA: MetaCreations Corp.

GoLive Cyberstudio 4.0 [Computer software]. San Jose, CA: Adobe Systems Inc.

HomePage 3.0 [Computer software]. (1998). Santa Clara, CA: FileMaker, Inc.

Meyen, E.L., Lian, C.H.T., & Tangen, P. (1997). Teaching on-line courses. *Focus on Autism and Other Developmental Disabilities, 12*(3), 166-174.

Office of Special Education Programs (1998). *Twentieth annual report to Congress on the implementation of the Individuals with Disabilities Education Act.* Washington, DC: U.S. Department of Education.

Photoshop 5.0 [Computer software]. (1998). San Jose, CA: Adobe Systems Inc.

Spooner, F., Spooner, M., Algozzine, B., & Jordan, L. (1998). Distance education and special education: Promises, practices, and potential pitfalls. *Teacher Education and Special Education, 21,* 121-131.

Curtis J. Bonk
Katrina Daytner
Gary Daytner
Vanessa Dennen
Steve Malikowski

Using Web-Based Cases to Enhance, Extend, and Transform Pre-Service Teacher Training: Two Years in Review

CURTIS J. BONK is Professor, Indiana University, Dept. of Counseling and Educational Psychology, School of Education, Room 4022, Bloomington, IN 47405-1006 (E-mail: CJBonk@indiana.edu).
KATRINA DAYTNER is Doctoral Student, Indiana University, Dept. of Counseling and Educational Psychology, School of Education, Room 4022, Bloomington, IN 47405-1006 (E-mail: kgilling@indiana.edu).
GARY DAYTNER is Doctoral Student, Indiana University, Dept. of Counseling and Educational Psychology, School of Education, Room 4022, Bloomington, IN 47405-1006 (E-mail: gdaytner@indiana.edu).
VANESSA DENNEN is Doctoral Student, Indiana University, Dept. of Instructional Systems Technology, Room 3044, Bloomington, IN 47405-1006 (E-mail: (vdennen@indiana.edu).
STEVE MALIKOWSKI is Doctoral Student, Indiana University, Dept. of Instructional Systems Technology, Room 3044, Bloomington, IN 47405-1006 (E-mail: smalikow@indiana.edu).

This paper was presented at the American Educational Research Association annual convention in Montreal, April 1999. Portions of the research presented here were funded by the Center for Global Change at Indiana University and by Proffitt Research Grant #29-402-01.

[Haworth co-indexing entry note]: "Using Web-Based Cases to Enhance, Extend, and Transform Pre-Service Teacher Training: Two Years in Review." Bonk, Curtis J. et al. Co-published simultaneously in *Computers in the Schools* (The Haworth Press, Inc.) Vol. 18, No. 1, 2001, pp. 189-211; and: *The Web in Higher Education: Assessing the Impact and Fulfilling the Potential* (ed: Cleborne D. Maddux, and D. LaMont Johnson) The Haworth Press, Inc., 2001, pp. 189-211. Single or multiple copies of this article are available for a fee from The Haworth Document Delivery Service [1-800-342-9678, 9:00 a.m. - 5:00 p.m. (EST). E-mail address: getinfo@haworthpressinc.com].

189

SUMMARY. This study was part of a two-year review regarding the use of Web-based case conferencing to enhance, extend, and transform the learning of pre-service teachers in an introductory educational psychology course. First, Web conferencing enhanced the learning opportunities within educational psychology by providing an electronically shared space for hundreds of students to share, discuss, and reflect on case situations common in K-12 school settings. Second, this environment extended learning by including students from other universities and countries. Finally, instead of strictly relying on instructor cases and commentary, the Web transformed the learning process by allowing students to generate cases online and provide timely and relevant peer feedback. Across the two years of this study, students generated more than a thousand case situations that tended to focus on classroom management, motivation, and controversial issues or hot topics. Within these case situations, students were extremely task focused and offered each other extensive peer feedback. Despite many positive findings, various problems were encountered such as procrastination, limited text referencing, and few justified statements. Several future directions and recommendations are outlined. *[Article copies available for a fee from The Haworth Document Delivery Service: 1-800-342-9678. E-mail address: <getinfo@haworthpressinc.com> Website: <http://www.HaworthPress.com> © 2001 by The Haworth Press, Inc. All rights reserved.]*

KEYWORDS. Asynchronous conferencing, teacher training, Web-based instruction, scaffolded instruction, e-learning, online mentoring, internalization, educational psychology, case-based learning, telecommunications

As educational technologies advance and the complexity of teaching intensifies, there is increasing attention regarding how technology can play a role in teacher education. Computer technology can be viewed as a tool to enhance, extend, or transform the teacher education curriculum. The project described here attempted to address all three of these important technology roles by using computer conferencing for more than two years in the teacher education curriculum. The creation of an electronic space for students to post and reflect on observed classroom case situations helped enhance the learning of hundreds of pre-service teachers. In terms of extending the learning environment, learning was electronically nurtured and coached by practicing teachers, instructors, and peers from around the world. While these mentors questioned ideas and suggested insights into solving various educational dilemmas, student learning was being extended to other locales. Finally, the center of control in the learning environment was transformed. Instead of discussing and solving case situations fabricated by the instructor, cases posted to the Web were constructed by the students based on actual experiences. Additionally, students discussed and debated how to resolve those dilemmas. As a result, these pre-service teachers were being prepared for the types of technology activities that they might later integrate into their own instruction.

CASE-BASED LEARNING

There is intense interest regarding how to make teacher education classes more meaningful through cases (Grant, 1992; Merseth, 1991; Richert, 1992; Silverman, Welty, & Lyon, 1992; Shulman, 1992). In addition to cases, some educators feel that early field experiences help contextualize key course concepts. A recent trend is the use of computer conferencing to create electronic discussion groups among pre-service teachers about topics of interest or problems seen in schools (Admiraal, Lockhorst, Wubbels, Korthagen, & Veen, 1997; Bonk, Malikowski, Angeli, & East, 1998). The project reported here combined all three of the above ideas and extended them one step further by using the Web as a tool for pre-service teachers to be apprenticed into the field of teaching with electronic mentoring from instructors, practitioners, and peers.

The first author has conducted a series of studies since the spring of 1997 to discover whether pre-service teacher Web-based conferencing about early field experiences can have a positive impact on pre-service teacher learning of educational psychology as well as their apprenticeship into teacher education. This research builds on an earlier comparison study of synchronous and asynchronous conferencing, favoring the latter (Bonk, Hansen, Grabner-Hagen, Lazar, & Mirabelli, 1998). However, instead of teacher-generated cases as in that first study, this particular set of studies used student-generated cases and an asynchronous Web-based conferencing. Here, students discussed such issues as inattentive students, teacher bias, and limited technology resources.

Since this project was situated within a Vygotskian or sociocultural camp (Wertsch, 1985; Vygotsky, 1978, 1986), we used the computer conferencing activity as a means for scaffolded feedback from a variety of learning participants. Several sociocultural scholars and researchers influenced the design of this learning activity. As part of an electronic apprenticeship (Rogoff, 1990), we attempted to build both vertical and horizontal mentoring with student case feedback coming from both peers and adult experts (Bonk, Malikowski, Angeli, & East, 1998). For example, students from other universities provided examples of similar situations they witnessed, whereas other instructors and expert teachers spoke from experience or posted a question intended to provoke discussion or reflection. Using the cognitive apprenticeship framework from Tharp and Gallimore (1988), we analyzed the forms of learning assistance taking place in these electronic discussions (Bonk, Malikowski, Angeli, & Supplee, 1998). From this perspective, we developed a template or guide sheet detailing a dozen ways to electronically mentor students (see Bonk, Hara, Dennen, Malikowski, & Supplee, 2000). The 12 forms of assistance in this template (e.g., direct instruction, modeling, scaffolding, pushing to explore or articulate ideas, etc.) (Bonk & Kim, 1998; Bonk & Sugar, 1998) varied greatly within the Web-based electronic conferences. For instance, while modeling was extremely limited in these online conferences, feedback and questioning were more common.

We believe that student-generated cases operate more readily within a student's zone of proximal development (ZPD) than prepackaged text cases or teacher-generated ones. By employing this approach, we hope that students internalize some of the strategies and recommendations they have encountered online with their peers and instructors. We also hypothesize that students' electronic conversations about their early field experiences will help them learn key course concepts; in effect, they should not only be able to recognize such concepts, but also to apply them when faced with similar situations. Along these same lines, semester-long conversations with other instructors, practicing teachers, and peers should enhance student ability to take the perspectives of others, while simultaneously helping them learn valuable technology skills.

Case-based learning on the Web may advance pre-service teachers' ability to take perspectives and internalize concepts. In effect, electronic conferencing in teacher education programs might help solve problems related to: (a) the isolation students feel when in the field; (b) the lack of community and dialogue among teacher education participants; (c) the disconnectedness between classroom knowledge and field experiences; (d) the limited reflective practices observed among novice teachers; and (e) the need to appreciate multiple perspectives and diverse cultures. In this project, more than one thousand different pre-service teachers electronically shared aspects of their field experiences over a five-semester span, while obtaining instructor and practitioner Web-based mentoring and feedback.

METHOD

Procedure

This summary research report stems from an extended study in pre-service teacher case-based discussions on the Web from the spring of 1997 to the spring of 1999. Most data analyses are of the first three semesters, however. Importantly, the tool for these case discussions, *"Conferencing on the Web"* or COW, remained the same throughout the project. Nevertheless, the number and level of participants, conference duration, and case topics varied each semester.

As a replacement for face-to-face discussions, pre-service teachers in this educational psychology course were asked to generate two teaching scenarios within COW based on problems or success stories that they viewed during their early field observations. Students were instructed to link theories and concepts from their class discussions and readings to their case observations. Writing and responding to these cases was a requirement of their 20-hour field experience. All names and places in these situations were to remain anonymous (Bonk et al., 2000; Bonk, Malikowski, Angeli, & East, 1998). The Web-based learning format of COW allowed students and instructors from multiple sections to comment on the cases posted. In many instances, teacher practitioners and teacher education experts provided comments and questions on these cases.

Students were asked to create two cases during the semester and respond to the case situations of six to eight peers. Within their own cases, students were to provide plausible resolutions for each case based on readings, lectures, and personal understandings (for a sample case, see Figure 1). The objective was to detail an interesting dilemma in terms of important concepts from one or more book chapters, and specify a personal recommendation for action in light of the course readings. Finally, students were to compare and reflect upon the differences between how they and the classroom teacher or textbook author might have resolved this dilemma. After posting their cases, students were typically asked to respond to Web cases of six to eight peers and, near the end of the conference, try to summarize the discussion within each of their own Web cases.

FIGURE 1. Sample Student Case in Conferencing on the Web (i.e., "COW")

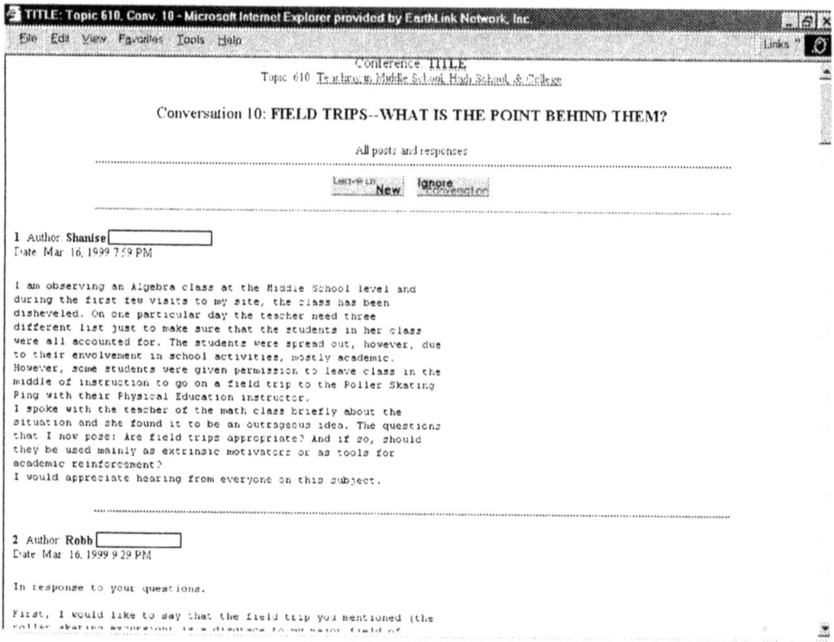

Participants

A large midwestern university coordinated the conference and Web server. Whereas most students and mentors were from this site, additional participants were located at other universities. In the first semester (spring of 1997), there were five sections of educational psychology generating and discussing cases; in the second semester (fall of 1997), there were six sections; and in the third semester (spring of 1998), there were three sections in the United States, and another 30 students from two universities in Finland. The latter semester included two full-motion videoconferences between the students in the United States and Finland–one at the start of the Web-based conferencing and one at the end. From the spring of 1997 through the fall of 1998, more than 700 students discussed their early field experiences using COW, creating more than 1,000 cases of elementary, middle school, and high school situations based on observations of actual teaching problems or dilemmas in the field.

Though not analyzed in much detail here, in the fall of 1998, there were approximately 300 students involving two universities in the

United States, two universities in Finland, and one university in Korea. In the spring of 1999, more than 100 students from another university in the U.S. as well as a few faculty and students from universities in Peru were added to the COW project. This group of nearly 400 participants created more than 600 cases. Across these semesters, there were often other students, instructors, graduate assistants, and practitioners who provided feedback to students and mentored them on their COW cases.

Quantitative Analyses

We have conducted a number of qualitative and quantitative analyses on the case data collected each semester. Only the quantitative data are reported here (for qualitative results, see Dennen & Bonk, 2000). For instance, the COW system logged all posting data, thereby enabling us to determine the total number of active participants, conference messages, and submitted cases. Through such data logging devices, we readily calculated the average length of discussion threads and cases, the average length of individual messages, the timing of student conferencing activities, and the depth of case discussion.

Across the first three semesters, 393 students generated a total of 687 cases or 1.75 cases per student. On average, then, we have had around 130 students using COW each semester to generate and discuss about 230 Web cases. From the spring of 1997 through the spring of 1998, there were a total of 3,832 messages, including 3,108 case replies, posted to the system. This equates to roughly 4.5 replies per case.

In comparison, in the fall of 1998, there were about 300 students involved from the U.S., Finland, and Korea. While the number of words per post fell to about 133 during this fourth semester of the COW project, there were 436 cases produced. Compared to typical case coverage of five to ten instructor cases per semester, such numbers are staggering! In total there were 2,491 messages in that conference of which 2,055 were case replies, which equates to approximately 4.7 replies per case. In the fifth semester (spring of 1999), the participants in the COW project continued to grow with additional students from the U.S. and Peru, though we had fewer participants from Korea and Finland. There were 624 cases posted in that semester and 1,768 replies or around 2.83 replies per case.

Interestingly, the average words per post increased each semester from 110 in the spring of 1997 to 130 in the fall of 1997 and then to nearly 140 in the spring of 1998. The words per post dipped slightly to 133 in the fall of 1998, but jumped to nearly 200 words in the spring of

1999. What elevated the discussion? This increase was likely due to better training, easier conference configurations, and the added international component. At the same time, the number of responses per case posted was reduced from around six responses per post in 1997 to three in 1999. In effect, while students engaged in greater depth of discussion, they did not respond within as many discussion threads.

Why is the raw data above important? Given that this was the first time most of these students actually traveled to a field experience, wrote a case, or corresponded using a Web-based conferencing tool like COW, this project was extremely successful at fostering student text production and social interaction. Students were engaged in a learning activity wherein they determined the topics of discussions and began offering advice as professionals in the field of teaching. They were engaged in a vibrant exchange of ideas across geographic locations and time. Students were extensively writing about common school experiences and receiving more feedback than typically experienced in conventional classroom settings. These and other findings are elaborated on and summarized at the end of this paper.

Case Evaluations

Portions of this conferencing data were previously analyzed to discover the forms of online mentoring, the depth of discussions, and student attitudes about the project (Bonk et al., 1998; Bonk, Malikowski, Supplee, & Angeli, 1998). To further evaluate the COW project and to begin construction of a public Web site of educational psychology cases, nearly 700 COW cases from the first three semesters of the COW project (i.e., Spring 1997, Fall 1997, and Spring 1998) were printed and rated. These cases were evaluated for quality, relevance, and topic(s) addressed. Information also was gathered regarding the grade level(s) and discipline(s) addressed by each case. Unfortunately, when students were writing their cases, they did not always specify the grade and/or discipline they were observing. In general, cases ranged across the K-12 spectrum and addressed all major disciplines–art, music, physical education, math, reading, English, foreign language, science, and social studies.

The selected cases were divided between two evaluators who rated their quality and relevance using two 3-point Likert scales. The *quality* scale included such categories as completeness, details, coherency, flow, and language use. The *relevance* scale, designed to evaluate the level of interest and debate commanded by each case, included ratings for interest, intrigue, uniqueness, relative importance, connectedness to course content, and controversy. This scale, in essence, asked, "Was this a hot topic?" Table 1 details these scoring rubrics.

Before coding the cases for this project, the two coders tested the coding rubrics on practice cases to determine the utility of the scales. Of the 687 total cases from the first three semesters of the project, 50 were coded by both raters to determine inter-rater agreement for each scale. For both raters, there was 80% agreement for both the quality and relevance scales. No rater differences were greater than one point.

DESCRIPTIVE RESULTS

Case Quality

Examination of case quality mean scores by semester revealed minimal variation; a score of two was given to a majority of the cases. Overall, students wrote cases that provided the reader with enough information to understand the situation being described and to understand the perspective of the observer.

Among the cases that did not receive a score of two or higher, the most common missing element was a lack of sufficient details or information necessary to fully understand the situation and foster student depth of processing. The reasons why these cases fell short may have included the limited number of field observations, time constraints, limited training in case construction, and a general lack of motivation to complete the task. In contrast, cases receiving a three were well-written from beginning to end and were full of details not only in regard to the events taking place, but also in relation to the contexts in which those events occurred. Such cases were detailed, meaningful, and important contributions to the learning community that the COW project attempted to foster.

Case Relevance

We calculated the average case relevance scores by semester. As was the case for the quality score, the majority of cases received a score of two for relevance. Highly relevant cases were written in a manner that peaked the interest of the reader by presenting situations that one could identify with and recognize as something he/she also observed or might likely encounter in the near future.

Cases receiving a low relevance score typically did not engage the reader. In such cases, the author typically failed to discuss a topic of general interest or wrote in a way that provided little meaning for the reader. Besides poor writing skills and time limitations, some cases were rated low as a result of students appearing to be interested only in receiving feedback for a specific situation, as opposed to providing a meaningful situation from which others could learn. Not surprisingly, cases rated high for relevance attracted the reader's attention from beginning to end with an intriguing situation; commonly these were cases that fostered the social and emotional development of students.

It is important to note that only a small percentage of cases made direct reference to course content and/or text content and thus this characteristic played a minimal role in rater coding for relevance. The lack of direct course or text reference may have been the result of students not yet mastering the course content at a level that would allow them to draw immediate connections to the situations they observed in their field placements. Also, since this was not a requirement for creating cases, students may have simply chosen to present what they observed for discussion (i.e., a contextualized story) without attempting to make connections to course content.

Total Case Scores

Total scores, ranging from two to six, were calculated by adding the quality and relevance scores for each case. A normal curve-like distribution was produced from the scores, with nearly one-half of the cases receiving a total score of 4. A score of 2 was given to 9% of the total cases; a score of 3 was given to 18% of the total cases; a score of 4 was given to 47% of the total cases; a score of 5 was given to 20% of the total cases, and a score of 6 was given to 6% of the total cases. The cases on the high end of these scales were primarily ones selected for inclusion in the Caseweb and INSITE projects, mentioned later, though they all required at least modest rewriting related to case contextualization and course connections.

Case Topics

As shown in Table 2, a wide variety of topics were discussed in the cases. Topic names were generated based upon the concepts and ideas addressed in typical introductory educational psychology textbooks (e.g., motivation, special education, classroom management, etc.).

TABLE 1. Coding Rubrics for Quality and Relevance Scales

Quality	1	*Completeness:* Lacks major components of case, serious omissions
		Details: Few or no essential and supporting details
		Coherency: Hard to follow, poor case structure
		Grammar: Poor sentence structure, several grammatical errors
	2	*Completeness:* Contains most but not all major components of case
		Details: Essential details present with few supporting details
		Coherency: Certain parts difficult to follow
		Grammar: Good sentence structure, some grammatical errors
	3	*Completeness:* All major components of case present
		Details: Essential details and supporting details present
		Coherency: Easy to follow from beginning to end
		Grammar: Good sentence structure, few or no grammatical errors
Relevance	1	*Interest:* Boring, trite, unoriginal
		Intrigue: Does not engage the reader
		Hot Topic: Not a current hot issue in the field
		Connection: Makes little or no connection to course content
		Controversy: Case content does not cause debate
	2	*Interest:* Generates some interest, shows some uniqueness
		Intrigue: Moderately engages the reader
		Hot Topic: A current or potentially hot issue in the field
		Connection: Makes some connection to course content
		Controversy: Case content is capable of starting debate
	3	*Interest:* Very interesting, rich examples, unique
		Intrigue: Highly engages the reader
		Hot Topic: A current hot issue in the field
		Connection: Makes some or many connections to course content
		Controversy: Case content sparks debate or multiple perspectives

Most cases discussed more than one topic, with more than 15 different major topics discussed overall. Knowing the issues that students were observing and finding interesting in schools helped us find certain types of cases to re-purpose for other uses.

By far, the most popular topic to write about was classroom management with approximately 312 cases of the 687 total related to that topic. Not surprisingly, the topic of management included both discipline and organizational matters such as physical environment of the classroom.

Why was management such a popular topic? It may be that students were concerned with how to manage their future classrooms and were looking for feedback regarding their observations. It could also be that management issues were the most obvious or explicit in student observations and included experiences found both within and outside of a classroom. Discussion of some of the other topics (development, for example) often required more interpretation and longer periods of observation.

In addition to management, students also chose to write a great deal about motivation (185 cases), instructional approaches (178 cases), and individual differences (152 cases). Again, it might be argued that students wrote about these topics more because they were concerned about how they might deal with these topics in the near future when they begin teaching. Some of our qualitative research detailed in other papers lends credence to these speculations (Bonk, Daytner, Daytner, Dennen, & Malikowski, 1999; Dennen & Bonk, 2000).

A unique and popular discussion area that emerged from the COW project was the "hot topic" category. This category did not necessarily reflect any particular idea or concept from the field of educational psy-

TABLE 2. Frequency of Topics Addressed in Cases

Topic	Number of Cases
Management	312
Motivation	185
Instructional Approaches	178
Individual Differences (special education and gifted)	152
Hot Topics (e.g., teacher burnout, violence in school, corporal punishment, and drugs and alcohol)	83
Development (physical, cognitive, and social/emotional)	70
Behaviorism and Social Learning Theory	57
Cognitive Processes (cognitive learning theories)	51
Assessment and Grading	37
Diversity and Group Differences	28
Teacher Behavior	22
Parents	20
Curriculum	17
Teacher Knowledge/Development	14
Technology	13

chology. Instead, this category encompassed global and controversial topics in education. Some examples of hot topics included teacher burn-out, parent-teacher relations, corporal punishment, drugs and alcohol, adolescent issues, teen suicide, violence in schools, and differences between the home and school. However, many students started posting cases to this area even when there was a relevant topic category already in COW that they should have utilized. The "hot topics" area was so popular, in fact, that by the start of the second semester, a notation had to be made to use this area only as a last resort.

Each semester, students were asked about their Web-based conferencing experiences. In these attitude surveys, students always found COW to be easy to use. The utility of the discussions and peer feedback, however, shifted during the first three semesters from mixed reviews to highly positive experiences. There are a few plausible reasons for this change including clearer directions, greater instructor modeling, and more authentic audiences in the conference such as the students from two universities in Finland. In fact, there are indicators that the addition of the international participants starting in the spring of 1998 raised the overall level and depth of discourse in COW.

OVERALL QUANTITATIVE FINDINGS

In summary, students wrote cases of average quality and relevance in each of the three semesters evaluated here. Overall, student case relevance scores were slightly higher than quality scores. While the total case quality and relevance scores of all 687 cases approximated a normal distribution, a wide variety of topics were discussed within these cases. The most popular topic was classroom management, followed by motivation, instructional approaches, and individual differences. At the same time, a unique set of hot topics emerged from the data that did not necessarily reflect a major topic or concept from the field of educational psychology, but that did encompass global and controversial topics in the field of education. Such controversial cases produced the most discussion.

It is important to note that the above findings fit prevailing learning and development theory. For instance, as both Piaget and Vygotsky would have expected, the controversial and unique cases (e.g., "What's the teacher for, anyway?," "Do computers replace teachers?," "My student and cocaine," and "Student plans to commit suicide") produced the most case dialogue. While student cases tended to gravitate toward classroom management and motivation issues, there also were a number of cases related to social issues (drugs, suicide) and religious concerns. The cases that encouraged responses had interesting contexts and problem situations, explicitly solicited student or instructor help, and were generally receptive to feedback.

As students become more familiar with using Web-based tools, the efficiency and ease with which they can be used as educational resources are increasing. There are a number of advantages associated with using COW as a resource for pre-service teachers conducting field observations. One advantage is that COW allows students to reflect on their field experiences prior to presenting their observations and ideas to others. Instead of a student attempting to jump into a classroom discussion and speaking with little forethought, one can organize his or her thoughts and present them in a coherent manner. This increases the meaning conveyed, while simultaneously enhancing the level of feedback.

Along these same lines, COW also allows individuals reading the cases to organize their thoughts prior to responding to their peers. There is time to think about the situation and the best ways to address it prior to responding. Such reflective responding can be a valuable component for students who do not like to react in a quick manner as well as for those who typically do not participate in classroom discussion. Additionally, COW is a valuable tool for students who are uncomfortable talking in class, since it provides an opportunity for students to talk to peers without the anxiety of speaking in front of a group. Consequently, such electronic experiences can be used as a bridge to move shy or introverted students to a more active role in class discussions.

Since students post their cases to a discussion forum, instructors can access the forum to see what issues their students are confronting in their field observations. Such access can be extremely beneficial when instructors lack sufficient class time to discuss student field experiences and concerns. Electronic conferencing is also beneficial when students go to their field observations at varying times and dates. Instructors can use time outside of class to discover how student observations are going as well as provide feedback and advice in an efficient and organized manner. Moreover, electronic conferencing offers a vital resource for those interested in seeing what common problems and issues are currently salient in K-12 classrooms.

In projects such as COW, students can read what other students are encountering during their field placements and hear how practicing teachers address a variety of tense and interesting situations. When students can compare how different teachers address similar situations, they are subsequently in a better position to think about how they might handle such situations when they are teachers. This capability is especially important for students who do not have many classmates from their major in class (e.g., speech and theater majors). As a result, students can learn from the experiences of their peers in other sections of the same course. In addition, students have an opportunity to discuss issues and ideas that are not addressed in the textbook or course lecture.

Computer conferences also provide students with a wealth of perspectives to draw upon. In addition to commentary and questions from peers and instructors, students can get feedback from teachers in the field or pre-service teachers observing in different contexts. Such individuals might supply examples of the classroom activities at both rural and urban schools as well as samples of how schools from other countries might be similar or different. When students organize responses in a written record or attempt to chronicle various opinions and ideas on a given situation, they begin to think about that situation from different perspectives instead of just one.

Finally, electronic collaboration with tools like COW not only provides a forum for discussion but also a resource for classroom instruction. For instance, an instructor might access interesting and relevant cases during class lectures or discussion to illustrate key concepts and ideas related to course content. Cases could be selected that address the concept of scaffolding or negative reinforcement. In effect, the instructor could use the electronic collaboration tools to provide a context in which students think about and understand course material.

MAJOR FINDINGS:
ENHANCING, EXTENDING, AND TRANSFORMING
STUDENT LEARNING WITH TECHNOLOGY

While there were admittedly some problems during the two and one-half years of the COW project, there also were several major accomplishments: for instance, Web-based conferencing using COW enhanced learning in the classroom by providing a vehicle for students to link concepts learned in class to actual school settings. In effect, the COW conference served as a safe harbor for these pre-service teachers to apply key terms and principles from their educational psychology textbooks. And instead of a few cases written and recycled by the classroom instructor, there were hundreds of cases for students to read, reflect upon, and debate, thereby further enhancing student learning.

As pointed out, we analyzed and rated the first three semesters of student work in COW. Using these ratings, we located and rewrote some of the most interesting and high quality cases. After linking these cases to different chapters of typical introductory educational psychology textbooks, we created the Caseweb site (see *http://www.indiana.edu/~caseweb*). The cases in the Caseweb included case introductions, questions, and sample feedback (see Figure 2). In addition, the cases were linked to a bulletin board system for students to discuss and debate from anywhere on the planet with an Internet connection. Students from various universities are now using the Caseweb for class discussions and quizzes, thereby further enhancing student opportunities to learn this material.

In addition to enhancing the learning of educational psychology, students in this project also learned about various educational technologies. For instance, COW participants grappled with how to use Web-conferencing technologies to communicate with other peers and instructors across the planet. In addition, a few students participated in videoconferencing experiences with Finnish students and instructors. Through these activities, hundreds of pre-service teachers learned how to structure electronic collaboration activities for their own technology-rich classrooms of the future. Student learning was clearly enhanced when we combined the pedagogical and technological aspects of the COW project.

Technology to Extend Learning

The COW project not only enhanced student learning, but also extended it beyond traditional classroom boundaries. Technology was utilized in the first two semesters of this project to enable students in one section of the educational psychology class to discuss their field experiences with students in other sections. Hence, their learning was extended beyond the single school that they were observing to the positive and negative experiences of peers in hundreds of other locales. Instructors, therefore, could compare and contrast the respective student field experiences, while students could see how key concepts played out in a myriad of real-life situations. Students who might otherwise have become depressed about their particular school or teaching situation perhaps began to realize that teacher work environments vary greatly.

FIGURE 2. The Caseweb Interface

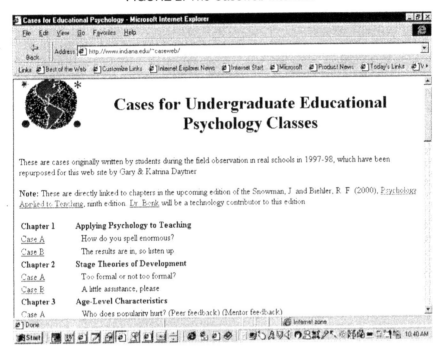

COW extended student learning beyond Midwestern K-12 settings to schools in other regions of the country as well as other continents. By the third semester, students from two Finnish universities were contributing and discussing cases in COW. In addition, during the fall of 1997 and spring of 1998, two videoconferences were held each semester for students to better understand one another. Further extending of the COW conference occurred when students from popular universities in Korea, Peru, and the southern U.S. were added to the COW discussions. In addition, practicing teachers and graduate students often provided pointed commentary and insightful questions on student case problems. Finally, during a couple of semesters, student teachers in international placements offered feedback and commentary from such locations as England, Australia, and Native American reservations. Such activities extend learning environments well beyond the normal educational psychology classroom.

International collaboration added a new dimension to the Web-based conferencing. As revealed in our qualitative research (Bonk, Daytner et al., 1999), students from Finland were older than the U.S. students and were more likely to back up their claims with citations to the relevant literature. Finnish student cases and case discussions were more in-depth, while instructor feedback was more horizontal or collegial in nature.

In effect, COW extended student learning to new and interesting places, while accumulating students' ideas in an electronic forum for later reflection and discussion. Unlike a traditional classroom wherein student oral contributions may soon be forgotten, in some classes, students were creating portfolios of their COW contributions–portfolios that might, in fact, stay with them throughout their undergraduate training and beyond.

Technology to Transform Learning

While COW was a legitimate tool to enhance and extend student learning, it also transformed it, if only for one course activity within a single semester. Nevertheless, since the spring of 1997, students in the COW project have constructed and debated more than a thousand cases about hundreds of different K-12 situations. As students socially negotiate meaning in COW, they gain a glimpse into how their peers and instructors might have solved certain problems and handled daily classroom dilemmas. In helping students co-construct this massive knowledge base of cases and responses, we were attempting to produce a learning community while promoting a different form of learning. To successfully participate in COW, it typically did not matter where you were physically located or when you wanted to join the learning community; COW was always awaiting your presence and participation.

Students in the COW conferences took some ownership over their learning and were constantly reflecting on situations that might arise when they began their professional careers. To foster ownership, the instructors assumed roles of coaches and consultants in this learning environment. Consequently, instructors and practicing teachers mentored student electronic learning by providing feedback, general recommendations, task structuring, pivotal questions, and indirect instruction. Such an approach is a transformation from the lecture-based instruction that often occurs in this type of course. At the same time, it aligns undergraduate educational psychology with the emerging social constructivist paradigm. In essence, COW instructors are practicing what they are preaching!

Other Findings: Pros and Cons

What else have we learned here? With minimal training, students readily adapt to the COW environment and generate hundreds of interesting cases in just a month or two of conferencing on the Web. Perhaps more importantly, the computer log data revealed that extensive feedback and advice on student teaching ideas occur long before students become certified teachers. On average, students receive four to five responses on their case situations. Equally important, off-task behaviors are minimal, as students are extremely task-focused and unaware of the quantity of electronic writing they produce. In COW surveys, students claim that the social exchange of these dilemmas helps confirm that the situations they are witnessing are indeed problematic and have many possible resolutions. Students especially like options to name their own topics, instead of relying on pre-established case categories (e.g., "Learning Styles" or "Assessment and Grading").

The interviews and surveys indicate that students benefit immensely from confirmation of ideas. With tools like COW, such confirmation and advice can come from instructors and mentors outside traditional classroom walls and scheduled meeting times. Here, students can be connected to others with parallel experiences. As a result, they can also receive feedback from peers who are interested in similar educational issues and problems. There is also more time for reflective and shy students to contribute to class discussions. And while class participation is less political, there are less disruptive and off-task behaviors than expected as students use tools like COW to complete a task. At the same time, there may be moments when it is important to encourage nonacademic discourse among participants since that builds opportunities for shared knowledge and the formation of learning communities.

Despite these positive findings, after more than two years of case conferencing, we still do not know how to transform this relatively brief, task-driven environment into an ongoing learning community. Too many students fail to obtain feedback on their cases because they procrastinate on case submission. Worse still, most case discussions lack sufficient justification or text referencing. Even though our interview data revealed that students believe that they retain more from the electronic conferencing, we do not yet have comparison data between Web conferencing students and those in traditional classroom settings. Further, while these discussions do not just happen automatically, it remains unclear how much structuring students require online as well as how to effectively manage masses of student input. When are electronic case discussions ever complete?

As indicated, a key problem here is that student discussion is primarily conversational and lacks appropriate relationships with course concepts and relevant literature. The fact that students simply want to post their stories and make comments based on personal experiences is not necessarily a negative finding; these initial conversations, in fact, may lead them on the road to teaching expertise. While students may also look at electronic conferences with preset requirements as busy work and an additional burden on their already busy schedules, the writing and reflection required by COW may have lasting impact. In fact, in the near future, we plan to develop case-based learning tools to further support student writing and reflection on the Web (for more details, see Bonk et al., 2000).

PEDAGOGICAL AND TECHNOLOGY RECOMMENDATIONS

Our experiences with COW lead to a number of technological and pedagogical suggestions. On the pedagogical side, instructors must create clear and user-friendly structures in electronic interactions (Bonk, Hara et al., in press). Such guidance is vital in lowering student anxiety and motivating students into Web-based learning. At the same time, instructors should not be hesitant to experiment with a variety of instructional techniques, some of which may not be highly structured or entirely clear, in attempts to foster both student interaction as well as personal reflection. Keep in mind that different conferencing tools can actually serve different instructional purposes. Tools for asynchronous or delayed collaboration like COW provide students with more time to reflect. But unlike the sequential conversational structure of COW, tools with threaded conversations allow students to send and receive more specific information and feedback.

Given the newness of the field of computer-supported collaborative learning, it is not surprising that there are a number of open issues and questions about the design of collaborative learning tools. In the near future, we envision Web sites like the Caseweb complete with directories of cases by subject area and topic. Embedded within those directories might be appropriate counter cases and case advisories from experts in the field. Sophisticated case tools might further include case introductions, expert commentaries, critical reviews, and associated video clips of different aspects of a situation. Ideally, students selecting a case would be allowed to view expanded or shrunken views, depending on the detail they require.

Sophisticated case tools might include the possibilities for labeling of case concepts and linking of key concepts between cases (Duffy, Dueber, & Hawley, 1998). To foster reflection, students might actually be forced to choose from a preset list of concepts before submitting their cases. Graphical link displays might show conceptual linkages across a series of cases or reference specific text segments from a case. To force more heated debate and controversy, there also is a need for role taking and mentoring options within the cases. In fact, with electronic cases, samples of previous mentor and peer feedback can be permanently stored for future learners. In this way, expert teaching and advice is not lost when one moves or retires. Sample mentoring options and questions might also be embedded to help experts and practitioners guide or mentor student learning. Finally, case comparison statistics can help users get a sense of the raw number of cases, most active topics and cases, range of feedback, depth of discussions, and timing of interactions.

For tools like COW and the Caseweb to flourish, electronic mentoring guidebooks and training programs need to be developed. In addition, online mentoring success stories might help those contemplating the use of online case-based learning.

FUTURE DIRECTIONS

Pilot tests of COW with modest funding have now touched over 1,000 students from 30 college classes who have electronically interacted with various peers, instructors, and practitioners. With additional funding, this project could reach tens of thousands of pre-service teachers around the world. Our research to date indicates that such electronic conferencing offers rich environments for students to share real-life teaching stories with peers and instructors.

Recently, we embarked on the next step of the COW project by creating *The Intraplanetary Teacher Learning Exchange* (TITLE), a place to connect pre-service teachers, instructors, and mentors across the globe, thereby enhancing the range of insight and advice on the Web related to teaching and learning. We also created a Web site called "INSITE" (see *http://college.hmco.com/education/insite/*) to support a popular educational psychology textbook, *Psychology Applied to Teaching*, published by Houghton Mifflin. INSITE contains cases, debates, field observation questions, classroom activities, and opportunities for instructors to share stories of teaching. Additionally, the tens of thousands of students reading this textbook can share their ideas related to a case situation or activity on the Web. Finally, we are developing a Web site entitled "CourseShare.com" with even more enhanced collaborative capabilities. Web resources such as TITLE, INSITE, and CourseShare.

com move beyond ways to enhance, extend, and transform the learning of a few hundred undergraduate teacher education students, to thinking about how tens of thousands of college instructors and students around the globe can create and collaborate on cases and other instructional activities.

We are just beginning to understand how pre-service teachers can find more meaningful connections to educational psychology through Web-based conferencing. Electronic cases can link multiple sections of the same course or similar courses in different countries for interesting cross-cultural discussions, debates, and collaborations. Overall, asynchronous Web-based conferences have tended to promote extensive social interaction and dialogue on early field experiences, timely instructor and expert mentoring wrapped around authentic problems, and vast amounts of text in this jointly shared electronic space. We hope you join us in exploring such unique and important electronic learning venues.

REFERENCES

Admiraal, W. F., Lockhorst, D., Wubbels, T., Korthagen, F. A. J., & Veen, W. (1997, August). *Computer-mediated communication in teacher education: Computer conferencing and the supervision of student teachers.* Paper presented at the 7th bi-annual meeting of the European Association for Research on Learning and Instruction, Athens, Greece.

Bonk, C. J., Daytner, K., Daytner, G., Dennen, V., & Malikowski, S. (1999, April). *Online mentoring of pre-service teachers with Web-based cases, conversations, and collaborations: Two years in review.* Paper presented at the American Educational Research Association annual convention, Montreal, Canada.

Bonk, C. J., Hansen, E. J., Grabner-Hagen, M. M., Lazar, S., & Mirabelli, C. (1998). Time to "connect": Synchronous and asynchronous case-based dialogue among pre-service teachers. In C. J. Bonk & K. S. King (Eds.), *Electronic collaborators: Learner-centered technologies for literacy, apprenticeship, and discourse* (pp. 289-314). Mahwah, NJ: Erlbaum.

Bonk, C. J., Hara, H., Dennen, V., Malikowski, S., & Supplee, L. (2000). We're in TITLE to dream: Envisioning a community of practice, "The Intraplanetary Teacher Learning Exchange." *CyberPsychology and Behavior, 3*(1), 25-39.

Bonk, C. J., & Kim, K. A. (1998). Extending sociocultural theory to adult learning. In M. C. Smith & T. Pourchot (Eds.), *Adult learning and development: Perspectives from educational psychology* (pp. 67-88). Mahwah, NJ: Erlbaum.

Bonk, C. J., Malikowski, S., Angeli, C., & East, J. (1998). Case-based conferencing for pre-service teaching education: Electronic discourse from the field. *Journal of Educational Computing Research, 19*(3), 267-304.

Bonk, C. J., Malikowski, S., Supplee, L., & Angeli, C. (1998, April). *Holy COW: Scaffolding case-based "Conferencing on the Web" with pre-service teachers.* Paper presented at the American Educational Research Association annual convention, San Diego, CA.

Bonk, C. J., & Sugar, W. A. (1998). Student role play in the World Forum: Analyses of an Arctic learning apprenticeship. *Interactive Learning Environments, 6*(1-2), 1-29.

Dennen, V., & Bonk, C. J. (2000). *Cases, conferencing, and communities of practice: A qualitative study of online mentoring for pre-service teachers.* Manuscript submitted for publication.

Duffy, T. M., Dueber, B., & Hawley, C. (1998). Critical thinking in a distributed environment: A pedagogical base for the design of conferencing systems. In C. J. Bonk & K. S. King (Eds.), *Electronic collaborators: Learner-centered technologies for literacy, apprenticeship, and discourse* (pp. 51-78). Mahwah, NJ: Erlbaum.

Grant, G. E. (1992). Using cases to develop teacher knowledge. In J. H. Shulman (Ed.), *Case methods in teacher education* (pp. 211-226). New York: Teachers College Press.

Merseth, K. K. (1991). The early history of case-based instruction: Insights from teacher education today. *Journal of Teacher Education, 42*(4), 263-272.

Richert, A. E. (1992). Writing cases: A vehicle for inquiry into the teaching process. In J. H. Shulman (Ed.), *Case methods in teacher education* (pp. 155-174). New York: Teachers College Press.

Shulman, L. S. (1992). Toward a pedagogy of cases. In J. H. Shulman (Ed.), *Case methods in teacher education* (pp. 1-30). New York: Teachers College Press.

Silverman, R., Welty, W. M., & Lyon, S. (1992). *Case studies for teacher problem solving.* New York: McGraw-Hill.

Tharp, R., & Gallimore, R. (1988). *Rousing minds to life: Teaching, learning, and schooling in a social context.* Cambridge, MA: Cambridge University Press.

Vygotsky, L. S. (1978). *Mind in society: The development of higher psychological processes* (edited by M. Cole, V. John-Steiner, S. Scribner, & E. Souberman). Cambridge, MA: Harvard University Press.

Vygotsky, L. (1986). *Thought and language* (rev. ed.). Cambridge, MA: MIT Press.

Wertsch, J. V. (1985). *Vygotsky and the social formation of the mind.* Cambridge, MA: Harvard University Press.

Douglas M. Harvey
Veronica M. Godshalk
William D. Milheim

Using Cognitive Flexibility Hypertext to Develop Sexual Harassment Cases

SUMMARY. The use of cognitive flexibility theory as a theoretical framework for designing hypertext has been found to be beneficial for learning in ill-structured domains. However, little is known of what role the learning *task* plays in the effectiveness of this approach. The present study examined the relationship between task, navigation, and learning transfer when utilizing a cognitive flexibility hypertext about sexual harassment with 34 graduate management students. Due to the nature of the topic, the effects of the task on student attitudes were also studied. The conclusions of the study were that there were no significant differences for the navigational choices or transfer

DOUGLAS M. HARVEY is Assistant Professor, Instructional Technology, The Richard Stockton College of New Jersey, P.O. Box 195, Pomona, NJ 08420 (E-mail: harveyd@loki.stockton.edu).
VERONICA M. GODSHALK is Assistant Professor of Management and Organization, The Pennsylvania State University, Penn State Great Valley, Malvern, PA 19355 (E-mail: vmg3@psu.edu).
WILLIAM D. MILHEIM is Associate Professor of Education, Instructional Systems, The Pennsylvania State University, Penn State Great Valley, Malvern, PA 19355 (E-mail: wdm2@psu.edu).

[Haworth co-indexing entry note]: "Using Cognitive Flexibility Hypertext to Develop Sexual Harassment Cases." Harvey, Douglas M., Veronica M. Godshalk, and William D. Milheim. Co-published simultaneously in *Computers in the Schools* (The Haworth Press, Inc.) Vol. 18, No. 1, 2001, pp. 213-229; and: *The Web in Higher Education: Assessing the Impact and Fulfilling the Potential* (ed: Cleborne D. Maddux, and D. LaMont Johnson) The Haworth Press, Inc., 2001, pp. 213-229. Single or multiple copies of this article are available for a fee from The Haworth Document Delivery Service [1-800-342-9678, 9:00 a.m. - 5:00 p.m. (EST). E-mail address: getinfo@haworthpressinc.com].

213

scores, but there did appear to be a relationship between task and changing students' attitudes towards the topic. *[Article copies available for a fee from The Haworth Document Delivery Service: 1-800-342-9678. E-mail address: <getinfo@ haworthpressinc.com> Website: <http://www.HaworthPress.com> © 2001 by The Haworth Press, Inc. All rights reserved.]*

KEYWORDS. Cognitive flexibility hypertext, navigation, task, sexual harassment

In the spring of 1999 the authors were involved in a project in which case studies, delivered using the World Wide Web (WWW), were used for instruction in a graduate management course on communication. As one of the course's experiential activities, hypertext materials were used to discuss issues of sexual harassment in the workplace. This article describes the theoretical rationale for using cognitive flexibility theory (Spiro, Vispoel, Schmitz, Samarapungavan, & Boerger, 1987) to guide the design of this hypertext system, the development process and implementation of the hypertext system, and the statistical analysis of the resulting assessment of student knowledge and understanding of the topic.

THEORETICAL RATIONALE

Cognitive flexibility theory (Spiro et al., 1987) maintains that instruction in ill-structured domains must allow the learner to "criss- cross" the domain knowledge so that the learner understands the interconnection of domain concepts and how the application of these concepts changes with the situation at hand. In other words, learners must be flexible in their understanding of a topic in order to apply important concepts appropriately in *any* given situation, not just those presented through the case study.

This differs in some important respects from the common use of a single, large case study. Specifically, the use of cognitive flexibility suggests the following:

1. A need for multiple case studies to insure that a variety of possible situations are presented.
2. A focus on cross-case differences in how concepts and principles are applied.

3. The use of concepts that are connected and applied across case scenarios as opposed to their presentation in a single case scenario.

According to Spiro and Jehng (1990), this "criss-crossing" connection of concepts and cases is most readily accomplished using the capability of hypertext systems (such as the World Wide Web) to explicitly link information. The key to deciding how to link concepts is to provide *themes* and *perspectives* that are common across the cases. In the present instructional setting, these themes and perspectives created a navigational system that learners were able to access and use to understand the nuances of the sexual harassment cases. In this manner, the students had access to a functional navigational system that was also integral to presenting the complexity of the domain knowledge.

By definition, *themes* are overarching concepts within the domain that are common to every context that may be encountered. Themes also act as an organizing framework for the cases and the concepts within a given instructional lesson. Within the hypertext designed for the sexual harassment module in the current course, themes such as power, responsibility, and societal views of sexual harassment were used to provide the common structure through which the learner examined the topic in all cases. In some manner all of the cases addressed issues relevant to all three themes.

In contrast, *perspectives* are the actors' viewpoints in the domain situations providing salient information about an individual case as well as a linking mechanism for learner exploration. For example, each of the sexual harassment situations had a group of actors including: (a) an alleged harasser, (b) an alleged victim, (c) a manager, and (d) at least one coworker. All actors were involved in the alleged sexual harassment in some way. The learner could mouse click between each actor's comments, gaining information about the case from the actor's viewpoint. In this way, the actor's viewpoints in each case could be compared with each of the other actors' viewpoints in each of the other cases.

In terms of navigation, the themes and perspectives enabled the learner's exploration of specific case information. Instructionally, this linking framework allowed learners to gain an understanding of the knowledge structure of the domain without sacrificing any complexity within it. In this way, material is not learned separately from the important domain concepts, but rather is understood to be interconnected and inseparable from the context-driven application of the concepts. Based on cognitive flexibility theory, this type of instruction should result in a more flexible understanding of the domain, which can then be readily applied at a later time in other domain situations that the learner may encounter.

While somewhat difficult to explain through a written narrative, operationalized cognitive flexibility is much more easily understood by viewing and interacting with an example. The specific hypertext system described in this article may be viewed at *http://www.higherweb. com/projects/cfh/*. At this Web site, you can login using the name "guest" and experience a learner's capability for navigating among the themes and perspectives in all cases or choosing instead to utilize one actor's viewpoint within a specific case.

DEVELOPMENT PROCESS

A team consisting of the course instructor, two instructional designers, and a Web-page developer was formed to design and create the hypertext materials. This section will describe the process used by the team to develop a cognitive flexibility hypertext on sexual harassment. The hypertext was primarily designed for teaching graduate management students the complex topic of sexual harassment and its potential impact in the corporate workplace.

Identification of Content and Themes

The first step was to examine the course objectives related to the activities where the hypertext would be used. In this activity, the students were to reflect upon their own understanding and biases regarding the issue of sexual harassment. The topic had been previously covered in the course through readings and discussion of a single case study.

The next concern of the instructional design group was to identify the themes and important concepts of the domain. Using a combination of the instructor's notes from previous lectures on the topic, and a similar set of hypertext-based case materials developed for use in an undergraduate course (Wyatt & Harvey, 1997), the team identified three themes and four perspectives for the sexual harassment content domain. The themes were power, societal views, and personal responsibility. The perspectives included the alleged victim, the alleged harasser, an involved coworker, and management. An additional perspective covering the legal views of sexual harassment was also considered important, since the part-time MBA students were adult learners working full time in corporate settings. All of these were then used as learning context guides during the development process.

Developing Case Studies

The instructional design team next sought to identify actual cases from legal articles and the popular press that clearly contained elements of all three themes. For example, one case involved a woman who was suing for harassment when a supervisor allegedly encouraged inappropriate, sexually explicit ridiculing of the female employee (power theme). Furthermore, several coworkers had suggested she was blowing the incident out of proportion (societal views). Another coworker stood by the woman, at some risk of ridicule to herself (personal responsibility).

The team determined that four cases were sufficient to show the breadth of the content domain in terms of possible scenarios, given the three-hour time frame available for the activity. The four cases involved:

1. A toy company executive who makes alleged sexual advances on a female sales representative.
2. A group of male employees who allegedly tease and make lewd comments to a female coworker.
3. A female office worker who alleges her supervisor established sexually harassing policies (i.e., what he thought was appropriate clothing for women in the workplace).
4. A male employee who alleges a female supervisor made unwelcome sexual advances toward him at a work site.

The information gathered on each case was used as the basis for writing case narratives. Fictitious names, companies, and hypothetical case specifics were inserted to create the content of each case. After the cases were written, they were incorporated into the hypertext system by the Web-page developer.

Designing the Hypertext System

A template was built for the actual hypertext system. Based on the tenets of cognitive flexibility theory, it was determined that maximum navigational "criss-crossing" of cases should be allowed, thus insuring that a learner would be able to jump from *any* page in the hypertext to nearly any other page in just one or two mouse clicks. The instructional screens were therefore formatted with links to each case available at the top of the screen, as well as links to both broad (themes and legal/policy links) and case-specific commentaries (themes and perspectives) on the left side. This design reserved the majority of the remaining space on each page for the case's text content.

Using this template design insured a strong interweaving of the cases, themes, and perspectives, allowing learners maximum flexibility in navigating the content. The template approach also simplified the process of importing the content into Web pages, since the development of each page required only input into the reserved space, with only minor changes in the case-specific links when necessary.

Integrating Content with the Hypertext System

The next step was to develop the content for the various hypertext pages. There were three levels of content:

1. *Themes.* Theme descriptions were designed to assist the learner with putting the case information into a broader framework of important domain concepts. Every character's viewpoint was designed to exemplify a particular theme in either a positive or negative way. For example, in one case the manager appeared to abuse his power; while in another, a manager was careful to follow company policy and to deal seriously with the woman's complaint.

2. *Case Narratives.* Narratives were designed to make the cases appealing and interesting, including using fictionalized characters (such as the manager involved). These characters provided a first-person account of the events and coworkers who described the situation facing the alleged victim from a different perspective. For each case, one page was devoted to describing the case, with links to each character as well as to the case-specific commentaries.

3. *Case Commentaries.* Commentaries for each case facilitated learner connections across themes, perspectives, and legal concepts, assisting the learner to consider the variety and complexity of the concepts at hand. In addition, objective legal information (such as applicable laws and a sample of the university policy on sexual harassment) was linked to emphasize the importance of the legal definition.

Once all content was written, the individual word-processed files were imported into the appropriate Web pages. For research purposes, JavaScript was included with each page to provide a tracking mechanism for learner navigation choices. The entire hypertext was then placed on a dedicated Web host server. After testing the hypertext to insure a properly functional system, the design and development of the technical system were complete.

Designing the Instructional Activity

To help promote learner engagement with the content (Jacobson, 1994), an instructional activity was deemed necessary. This required the development of a compelling reason for the learner to want to use the hypertext to explore this issue (sexual harassment). Based on this requirement, we asked the learner to assume the role of either a juror deciding on each case or a human resources manager developing a policy for his or her company. It was our intention that either of these tasks would be sufficient to motivate the learners in their examination of the cases in order to make informed decisions in the completion of their assignment.

Summarizing the Development Process

In summary, the process used to design and develop the cognitive flexibility hypertext system involved:

1. Defining themes and perspectives important to the domain.
2. Developing realistic cases that involved themes, perspectives, and commentaries.
3. Producing hypertext structure that allowed the "criss-crossing" of cases.
4. Writing and importing content into the hypertext structure.
5. Designing engaging tasks to facilitate the use of the hypertext system by its intended audience.

The outcome of this process was a 2- to 3-hour instructional activity in which students were instructed to view a cognitive flexibility hypertext with the goal of accomplishing their assigned task (either developing a verdict or writing an appropriate policy).

IMPLEMENTATION

The hypertext activity was implemented with two sections of a graduate management course concerning communications in the workplace. One course section was taught in a face-to-face lecture format, while the other was offered online, utilizing FirstClass conferencing software and e-mail for instructor-student and student-student interactions. The hypertext activity was used with both sections, although implementation was slightly different for the online course.

The face-to-face section devoted a normal three-hour class to the experiential activity. This class of 22 students was instructed to use computers in a public computer lab reserved for the class activity. First, the students were asked to complete a 16-item attitudinal questionnaire regarding sexual harassment (Appendix A), instructed how to access the hypertext system on the WWW, and randomly assigned to one of the tasks (policy creation or juror decision) embedded within it. All students were also asked to write down the time that they started and the time they completed the activity.

Once students logged on to the site, they were allowed to explore the hypertext materials at their own pace and to view pages in whatever order they wished. The instructor and other members of the design team were available for help with technical problems or to answer questions regarding the assignment.

In addition, students were encouraged to take advantage of other computing resources by opening a word-processing program in addition to the hypertext Web site, which enabled them to complete the written portion of their assignment as they utilized the hypertext. After students completed the assignment, they were instructed to turn in their written verdict or policy to the instructor before leaving the lab.

One week after completing the hypertext activity and assignment, each student in the face-to-face group was asked to complete the sexual harassment attitude survey a second time, just prior to taking the final exam for the course. The final exam was administered in a three-hour session as part of the final class meeting. Within the final exam, there were two questions in which the student was presented with a short paragraph describing a potential sexual harassment case and asked to provide a decision regarding whether the situation involved sexual harassment. A third answer option was that there was not enough information to make a determination. For any of the three answers provided, the student was required to provide a rationale for his or her decision.

In contrast, the 14 students in the distance-education section of the course were given the same activities and assignments via asynchronous means. As with the face-to-face students, the students were randomly assigned to one of the two activities, with seven students in each group. The sexual harassment attitude survey was mailed to each student one week prior to beginning the activity. After all surveys were returned, an e-mail message was sent to each student with instructions for logging on to the WWW site and the description of the hypertext activity. After completing the assignment, each online student sent his or her answers in an electronic text message to the instructor.

The online students were assessed at distance, as opposed to taking the final exam in a face-to-face setting, with the follow-up sexual harassment questionnaire sent to all of these students along with their final exam. After completing the questionnaire, students were instructed to complete the exam, which included the two questions regarding sexual harassment. Students had several days in which to complete the exam, after which they were to send the survey and exam to the instructor.

While there were some differences in the methods used with each section, we believe that the face-to-face and online students had very similar experiences utilizing the hypertext system.

ASSESSMENT AND EVALUATION

After gathering the navigational data and the student answers, the design team coded and analyzed the information to examine the possible interrelationships among navigation, transfer of knowledge, and attitude. In other words, the analyses were an attempt to discover whether the use of cognitive flexibility theory as a framework for developing and using hypertext materials would prove advantageous for (a) understanding the concept of sexual harassment, (b) learning the nuances associated with the definition of sexual harassment, (c) understanding U. S. laws pertaining to sexual harassment issues, and (d) understanding the complexity of the issue as it relates to corporate policies and implementation.

Navigation

Based upon the theoretical concept of criss-crossing proposed by Spiro et al. (1987), the navigational data were examined to determine whether students had jumped between case and theme information while using the hypertext. In terms of this variable, students appeared to criss-cross at a relatively low rate regardless of whether they were assigned the juror task (Mean = 11.82, SD = 8.01, n = 17), or the policy-making task (Mean = 8.24, SD = 8.47, n = 17). Students therefore viewed each case separately and looked at all the pages associated with the current case before moving to the next one. There was only a small amount of evidence to suggest that students were engaged in the type of reviewing and juxtaposition of case and theme information that the theory suggested.

Further inspection of the data, using an independent samples t-test, revealed that the assigned task, either jury (n = 17) or policy (n = 17), had no statistically significant impact on navigational choices (t = -1.269, df = 32, $Sig.$ = .214, p > .05). However, in comparing the class sections, course environment (face-to-face versus online) was significantly related to the total amount of criss-crossing choices made, as revealed through calculating the Pearson correlation between class type and criss-crossing (r = .34, p < .05). The data suggests that participants in the online class did less criss-crossing than their counterparts in the face-to-face class.

One possible explanation for this difference in navigation by class section may be that the online students reported spending less time on the hypertext activity (Mean = 91 minutes) compared to the face-to-face students (Mean = 135 minutes). In other words, online students simply did not take as much time to make various criss-crossing choices. A 2 × 2 factorial analysis of covariance (ANCOVA), using time on task as a covariate (see Table 1), showed that if time is factored out, there are no statistically significant differences between navigation and task (F = 1.07, p > .05, n = 34) or navigation and class section (F = .356, p > .05, n = 34).

The overall conclusions related to navigational choice suggest that there was no clear relationship between the students' assigned task or class section and the way they navigated the hypertext system. Therefore, the amount of learner criss-crossing did not appear to be a function of task or environment, but of some other uncontrolled factor, such as time spent on the task.

Transfer of Knowledge

Three independent raters rated the transfer question essays according to a five-point rubric. For each question, raters were to consider the learner's application of the legal standards, thematic issues, and the interrelations between legal and thematic issues, and how detailed the answer was in providing a rationale. The final transfer score for each

TABLE 1. ANCOVA Table for Analysis of Task and Class Type Effects on Navigation Style with Time on Task as a Covariate

Source		SS	DF	MS	F	p
Between		193.478	3			
	Task	65.603	1	65.603	1.070	0.309
	Class	21.829	1	21.829	0.356	0.555
	Task*Class	106.046	1	106.046	1.730	0.199
Covariate						
	Time	55.328	1	55.328	0.903	0.350
Error		1777.808	29	61.304		
Total		2026.614	33			

learner was the combined total points for each question, with a maximum possible score of 10 points. Interrater reliability for the transfer scoring was 91.8% between raters 2 and 3; 91% between raters 1 and 3; and 93% between raters 1 and 2.

The resulting scores showed that students in the juror group (Mean = 4.79, SD = 1.58, n = 17) and students in the policy group (Mean = 5.13, SD = 1.82, n = 17) scored roughly the same on transferring what they learned to the new situations presented in the test. This suggests that the task assignment did not impact how much students learned or were able to apply from the material presented in the hypertext.

However, after calculating two-way Pearson product-moment correlation coefficients between class type and transfer scores, it was revealed that class type did appear to be significantly related to transfer of knowledge (r = .461, p < .01, n = 34). Inspection of the data revealed that the face-to-face group (Mean = 4.39, SD = 1.59, n = 22) scored lower than the online group (Mean = 6.00, SD = 1.37, n = 12). This may be explained by the differences between the type of class and the testing conditions, since face-to-face students completed the transfer questions as part of a timed exam in class, while distance students were allowed to take the same exam at home with no time limit. It is therefore possible that distance students scored higher on the transfer questions simply due to their having more time to answer the questions.

Having determined the transfer scores, a regression analysis of the total criss-crossing score showed no significant effect between navigational criss-crossing and transfer of knowledge (F = .083, p > .05, n = 34). A multiple regression on transfer of knowledge, using class type as a factor, was also run to determine if class type was obscuring the relationship between criss-crossing and transfer. The multiple regression revealed that neither class ($F = .095, p > .05$) or criss-crossing ($F = .083, p > .05$) played a significant role in the transfer scores. There was, therefore, no relationship between the total number of times that a student criss-crossed the hypertext and the transfer of knowledge as measured by the essay questions.

The final option related to knowledge transfer was that assigned task might show a significant impact on transfer due to the relationship between the task and the student's navigation style. A 2 × 2 blocked ANOVA (see Table 2) was conducted on transfer scores, using task type as the independent variable, and class type as a blocking factor. This showed that task still had no significant relationship to transfer ($F = .350$, $p > .05$, $n = 34$). While this study is exploratory with a small sample size, these results lead to a tentative conclusion that there were no apparent effects regarding task, navigation, and transfer from using the hypertext activity with the students.

Attitudes

Attitude regarding sexual harassment was measured via a questionnaire (see Appendix A) prior to the instructional treatments and again prior to the transfer test. Beauvis (1986) considered attitude to be a combination of knowledge, sensitivity, and awareness of the issue of sexual harassment. In the present situation, the method for measuring the change in pre- and post-treatment sexual harassment attitudes was twofold. First, participant answers were compared with those of an outside expert who was highly knowledgeable regarding the issue of sex-

TABLE 2. ANOVA Table for Analysis of Task Type on Transfer Score with Class Section as a Blocking Factor

Source	SS	df	MS	F	p
Between	24.854	3			
Task	2.020	1	2.020	0.862	0.361
Class	20.029	1	20.029	8.543	0.007
Task X Class	2.805	1	2.805	1.196	0.283
Within	70.337	30	2.345		
Total	95.191	33			

ual harassment. A perfect score for the questionnaire was 16 (every answer matching the expert). An answer that matched the expert's was given one point, with the resulting total score used for statistical analysis. Second, pre- and post-treatment attitude scores were compared to assess the learner's change in attitude. These scores were then used as the basis for statistical analysis of this change to determine if task type had any impact on attitudes about sexual harassment.

A repeated measure statistical analysis was conducted using a two-way, 2×2 factorial ANOVA, with type of task as the independent variable and pre-test and post-test attitude scores as the dependent variable. This analysis revealed that there was a significant interaction between pre-activity to post-activity attitude survey scores and the type of task ($F = 4.86, DF = 1,33, MS = 2.431, p < .05$). Inspection of the data revealed that the policy task group ($n = 16$) showed a mean positive change of 1.25 points on the attitude survey from pre-activity to post-activity, while the juror task group ($n = 17$) had a mean negative change of -0.41 (see Figure 1). This meant that students from the policy task group evidenced attitudes that, after the instructional activity, were more like those of an expert who is very aware and sensitive to the issue of sexual harassment.

This finding leaves us with the possibility that the type of assignment, although not impacting the transfer of knowledge, may have played a role in the students' change of attitude toward the topic of sexual harassment.

FIGURE 1. Differences in Pre- and Post-Test Scores on Sexual Harassment Questionnaire Grouped by Task Type

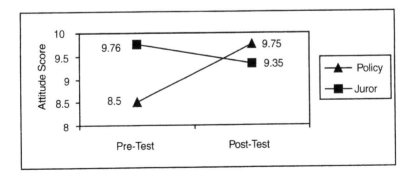

RESEARCH IMPLICATIONS

While the results of the study did not yield the expected significant differences in terms of knowledge transfer, they do suggest some reasons to consider altering our use of cognitive flexibility hypertexts when the domain involves *affective* components, as was the case with sexual harassment in this study. Specifically, the nature of the learning tasks that are provided to help guide learners in their use of hypertext may impact the attitudes of these learners about the topic.

When dealing with domains that involve strong emotional, and perhaps controversial opinions, the task may need to be designed so that learners remain open to the complexity and ill-structured nature of the knowledge being represented. In the present case, it appeared that a task requiring learners to merely indirectly state their preconceived opinions (through a policy decision) was able to facilitate the affective goals of the instruction better than a task that forced learners to make correct or incorrect decisions (as is the task of juror).

Beauvis (1986) notes that sexual harassment training is designed to change attitudes by challenging trainees' opinions on the issue. The goal is to make participants more aware and more sensitive, which means they may need to be exposed to information that is contradictory to their beliefs. In explaining the results of our use of a cognitive flexibility hypertext, it seems reasonable that perhaps the two tasks (jury versus policy) were different in how participants interacted with contradictory viewpoints on sexual harassment. Learners asked to provide a verdict in each case were perhaps more likely to hold on to their beliefs in the face of new information, since they were stating and defending their personal opinions in light of legal standards. This could be construed to mean they were forced to either accept or reject new information, or to reinterpret the information on the basis of their personal understanding regarding sexual harassment law.

On the other hand, the learners developing policy may have been taking a more open perspective on the information they encountered, since developing a comprehensive policy meant taking into account as many different possibilities and perspectives as possible. In order to do this, these learners may have been acting less on personal belief than those in the jury group, and therefore they were more willing to accommodate information that contradicted their beliefs.

All of these changes to the structure of the current research study present opportunities for future research. Another opportunity may be to test the operational definition of the term *criss-crossed*. According to Spiro et al. (1987), criss-crossing involves revisiting and juxtaposing case information. In this study, the statistical analyses were based on criss-crossing being operationalized as linking *between* cases and returning to a previously viewed case. In other words, learners had to jump from the content of one case to another case in order to have implemented the criss-crossing construct. This definition assumes that such navigational choices indicate the type of cognitive activity (review and juxtaposing information) called for in cognitive flexibility theory. However, it may be that learners *criss-cross content information* (themes and perspectives commentaries) *within a case*, and retain and apply that information as they move to another case. Since our navigational tracking system was in its infancy, future research may look not only at the navigational tracking system, but also at effect differences in between-case and within-case learner criss-crossing.

CONCLUSION

Since ill-structured domains tend to involve a great degree of variability with no true right or wrong answers, this study may suggest a new direction for studying cognitive flexibility theory. Findings of previous cognitive flexibility hypertext research examined beliefs regarding the nature of knowledge (Jacobson & Spiro, 1995; Jacobson, Maouri, Mishra, & Kolar, 1996), but not specifically the nature of the domain being studied. For ill-structured domains in which the learning outcomes may be affective (domains such as ethics, sociology, etc.), it may be that the nature of the task could play a significant role in learning by virtue of how the learner approaches information contradictory to his or her beliefs.

In conclusion, the use of cognitive flexibility theory appears to hold promise for improving instruction that involves affective components. In practical terms, it is important to insure that the task will prompt students' consideration of multiple perspectives, and challenge students' beliefs and assumptions. While previous studies of cognitive flexibility hypertexts have shown benefits for transfer of knowledge in nonaffective domains, it may be that such an approach can be equally useful for meeting affective outcomes.

REFERENCES

Beauvis, K. (1986). Workshops to combat sexual harassment: A case study of changing attitudes. *Signs: Journal of Women in Culture and Society, 12*(1), 120-145.

Jacobson, M. J. (1994). Issues in hypertext and hypermedia research: Toward a framework for linking theory-to-design. *Journal of Educational Multimedia and Hypermedia, 3*(2), 141-154.

Jacobson, M. J., Maouri, C., Mishra, P., & Kolar, C. (1996). Learning with hypertext learning environments: Theory, design, and research. *Journal of Educational Multimedia and Hypermedia, 5*(3/4), 239-281.

Jacobson, M. J., & Spiro, R. J. (1995). Hypertext learning environments, cognitive flexibility, and the transfer of complex knowledge: An empirical investigation. *Journal of Educational Computing Research, 12*(4), 301-333.

Spiro, R. J., & Jehng, J. C. (1990). Cognitive flexibility and hypertext: Theory and technology for the nonlinear and multidimensional traversal of complex subject matter. In D. Nix & R. J. Spiro (Eds.), *Cognition, education, and multimedia: Exploring ideas in high technology* (pp. 163-205). Hillsdale, NJ: Lawrence Erlbaum.

Spiro, R. J., Vispoel, W. P., Schmitz, J. G., Samarapungavan, A., & Boerger, A. E. (1987). Knowledge acquisition for application: Cognitive flexibility and transfer in complex content domains. In B. K. Britton & S. M. Glynn (Eds.), *Executive control processes in reading* (pp. 177-199). Hillsdale, NJ: Lawrence Erlbaum.

Wyatt, N., & Harvey, D. (1997, June). *Hypertext sexual harassment Web page.* Paper presented at the Ed-Media/Ed-Telecom conference sponsored by the Association for the Advancement of Computing in Education, Calgary, Alberta, Canada.

APPENDIX A
Sexual Harassment Attitude Questionnaire

Instructions: Rate statements 1-16 on a five-point Likert scale, from "strongly disagree" to "strongly agree," based upon the degree to which you feel the statement is true. Place an "X" in the box corresponding to your answer for each item.

	Strongly Agree	Agree	Not Sure	Disagree	Strongly Disagree
1. Sexual harassment rarely occurs.					
2. Sexual harassment is a violation of state law.					
3. One of the problems with sexual harassment is that some women can't take a joke.					
4. Sexual harassment can happen to men.					
5. People who are sexually harassed usually invite it.					
6. Few women are actually forced to change employment because of sexual harassment.					
7. Once a person becomes involved in a sexual relationship, he/she cannot allege sexual harassment.					
8. Homosexuals may be sexually harassed by persons of either sex.					
9. Women who wear provocative clothing are inviting a sexual response.					
10. Many charges of sexual harassment are frivolous and vindictive.					
11. Most incidents of sexual harassment are reported.					
12. Women who complain of sexual harassment are more often punished than the men who harass them.					
13. Women who are sexually harassed feel a great deal of shame and guilt.					
14. Issues of sexual harassment make it difficult for men and women to date.					
15. Sexual harassment has little to do with power.					
16. Managers and supervisors should refrain from dating their subordinates.					

Lucio Teles
Mary Ann Gillies
Stacy Ashton

A Case Study
in Online Classroom Interaction
to Enhance Graduate Instruction
in English Literature

SUMMARY. This paper discusses the use of online classroom collaborative environments to support the face-to-face teaching of a graduate course in English Literature. Online data from graduate students and the professor were collected and analyzed. Results show that students benefit from the online interaction to learn English Literature. There are, however, also disadvantages in the use of online environments, which are discussed in our conclusion. *[Article copies available for a fee from The Haworth Document Delivery Service: 1-800-342-9678. E-mail address: <getinfo@haworthpressinc.com> Website: <http://www.HaworthPress.com>* © 2001 by The Haworth Press, Inc. All rights reserved.]

KEYWORDS. Online education, English literature, higher education, educational technology

LUCIO TELES is Director, Centre for Distance Education, 8888 University Drive, Simon Fraser University, Burnaby, British Columbia V5A 1S6 (E-mail: teles@sfu.ca).
MARY ANN GILLIES is Associate Professor, Department of English, Simon Fraser University, Burnaby, British Columbia V5A 1S6 (E-mail: gillies@sfu.ca).
STACY ASHTON is Research Assistant, Department of Education, Simon Fraser University, Burnaby, British Columbia V5A 1S6 (E-mail: sashton@sfu.ca).

[Haworth co-indexing entry note]: "A Case Study in Online Classroom Interaction to Enhance Graduate Instruction in English Literature." Teles, Lucio, Mary Ann Gillies, and Stacy Ashton. Co-published simultaneously in *Computers in the Schools* (The Haworth Press. Inc.) Vol. 18. No. 1, 2001. pp. 231-248; and: *The Web in Higher Education: Assessing the Impact and Fulfilling the Potential* (ed: Cleborne D. Maddux, and D. LaMont Johnson) The Haworth Press, Inc., 2001, pp. 231-248. Single or multiple copies of this article are available for a fee from The Haworth Document Delivery Service [1-800-342-9678, 9:00 a.m. - 5:00 p.m. (EST). E-mail address: getinfo@haworthpressinc.com].

231

The impact of online educational technology and the online class-room in higher education has had many differential effects. While some areas that require the use of computers such as Departments of Computer Sciences, Biology, Administration, and others are benefiting from an increased student interest in taking their programs, other departments have not yet experienced a substantial change.

Departments of English Literature have reacted in different ways to the new challenge. While for some Departments of English Literature economic conditions are improving, English instructors are still generally being asked to do ever more with less. At the undergraduate level, many fear that the quality of their teaching is being sacrificed to the demand to process more students through heavier course loads and larger classes, with the concomitant increases in grading and student contact hours (Moran, 1993).

Economic pressure is also being felt in graduate programs. However, because graduate programs have a much smaller enrollment than undergraduate programs, the economies of scale sought out at the undergraduate level through the use of large classes and lectures are not available. One outcome of requiring relatively large class sizes (e.g., over six students) at the graduate level is under-enrollment and course cancellation. The marriage of fiscal economy and a necessarily small class size is a conundrum for administrators. This paper discusses one way in which this conundrum was dealt with by the Department of English Literature and describes a pedagogical response using online technology.

COURSE DESCRIPTION
AND CONTEXT OF DEVELOPMENT

In the fall of 1996, members of the Department of English Literature agreed to experiment with the way in which they taught graduate courses. The catalyst for this decision arose from a complex interaction of factors, as do all administrative decisions. An initial factor was student dissatisfaction with the number and topics of courses being offered each term. This university offers courses year round with a trimester system of three 13-week terms, and the English department typically offered three graduate courses in each of the fall and spring terms, and one in the summer term. Students acted on their dissatisfaction by cutting back their enrollment from two courses per term to one, in the hopes that the range and perceived attractiveness of course offerings would improve in future terms. The lower enrollment rate meant that many courses failed to reach minimum enrollment requirements, which led to fewer courses actually being offered. This trend led to increased dissatisfaction among students and faculty, whose teaching assignments were often changed at the last minute, creating a fair amount of administrative and personal chaos. At the same time, budget constraints ruled out the possibility of adding traditionally formatted courses or lowering the minimum enrollment requirement for existing courses.

The solution proposed to this dilemma involved extensive changes to the traditional course format. In the traditional model for graduate courses, students and instructors met weekly for five hours, and a combination of lecture, presentations, and discussions was the norm. Students received five credits for the course; faculty counted it as part of their regular teaching load. The Graduate Committee's new format involved offering at least four courses per semester with enrollment in each capped at six. Classes would meet for only two hours a week, so students would have to do substantial out-of-class work in order to earn the five credits assigned. Faculty would teach the courses in addition to their regular course load, and they would be entitled to a course release once they had taught two of these new courses. In addition, small groups of students would be encouraged to approach faculty to request courses on topics of mutual interest, thus ensuring enrollment. Although not all faculty were happy with this new system, and some opted not to be involved because they opposed extra-load teaching, the department launched the new format in the spring of 1997.

Pedagogical Response

Students were to take additional outside work to offset the decreased number of classroom hours. The challenge for the instructors was to identify designs that would deliver the same quality of instruction and intellectual engagement students have in longer classes while at the same time staying within the reduced instructional workload allotted by the new format. A potential solution was to enhance class discussion by using online peer collaborative environments, with the ongoing support of the instructor.

This solution was applied by the first author to the teaching of a graduate course titled "Material Modernism," dealing with early 20th century British literature (English 803), a topic initiated by students. The specific objective was to introduce online teaching in response to the current economic pressure; to explore options for redesigning a literature course with a different format, relying on active student participation and collaboration while still retaining the discussion mode central to such courses. We further hoped that in the long run such technology would lessen the growing burdens on individual instructors.

The use of asynchronous (i.e., not real time) online discussion to enhance instruction is being adopted quite widely in higher education (Bump, 1990). This approach has profound impact because students are expected to take a more active role in the learning process and instructors must learn new instructional skills (Harasim, Hiltz, Teles, & Turoff, 1995; Hiltz, 1994). Given the student-initiated nature of this course, the use of a technological platform designed to increase student activity and responsibility was considered appropriate.

The use of new pedagogical approaches via multimedia network technologies has been a focus of research at our university. One of our teams has created an online learning environment called Virtual-U (V-U). V-U is a conferencing tool for online courses that operates on a Web browser and offers asynchronous communication that allows students and instructors to discuss course materials and issues online. Asynchronous discussion is much like the e-mail technology with which most of us are now familiar. The participants post a message to the V-U class conference space and return to the conference later to check for responses from classmates or the instructor.

We saw V-U as a way to promote knowledge building by encouraging collaboration and information sharing outside of the limits of a two-hour class. The small class size in this course (four enrolled out of a maximum enrollment of six) was perceived as an ideal way to facilitate the instructor's process in learning to teach online while at the same time making it possible to offer student access to the department lab in order to avoid restricting the course to students who owned computers. The course was launched in January 1997.

Instructional Design of English 803

Two important goals were used to guide the design of the new version of English 803: the first was to make the best use of a mixed and online mode of teaching; and the second, to integrate the learning that occurred online with that during the in-class meeting. The vision for the course was to initiate a discussion loop between the physical and virtual classrooms, so that material posted online would be built upon in the face-to-face meetings, which would be further discussed online, and again in the next class, with each week's reading contributing more fuel to the ongoing conversation.

A learner-centered model was chosen for both the face-to-face meetings and the online conferences. The instructor deliberately chose to avoid lecturing in the face-to-face meetings, partly from a belief that the graduate level learning should be collaborative, and partly to maximize the opportunity for students to discuss the week's readings and issues arising from them. Students were expected to study in both modes, with the instructor acting as a facilitator. The instructor provided information, moderated the discussion, gave feedback, and pointed to appropriate texts related to the course discussion, but the onus was on students to run the classroom and online discussions.

The online conference component of the course had five areas for interaction: (a) Summary, in which class members were to place summaries of the week's reading assignments; (b) Readings, in which students could raise further points about any of the weekly readings or about issues raised in class discussion; (c) Research, in which students could discuss the nature and progress of their research projects for the course; (d) Help, for mutual help among students; and (e) Café, where students had a forum for the kind of end-of-class or coffee break chat that is often a feature of face-to-face courses. The five areas were separated because previous experience with V-U had demonstrated that, without some kind of segmentation, it became almost impossible to follow the thread of discussions generated by online conversation.

Each week prior to class meeting the four students and the instructor posted summaries of the assigned readings. Whenever possible, the instructor posted her own summaries after the students has posted theirs in order to avoid influencing the students' impressions. The weekly summaries were the mechanism by which the students and the instructor discussed the course material online. Making a connection between new and old readings was encouraged explicitly by the instructor as part of the criteria for a good summary.

The in-class discussions were also in large part shaped by the online summaries and discussions. Each week, one class member was assigned to lead off class discussion by providing a brief response to the online postings. This approach was intended to ensure that online discussion was integrated into the face-to-face meetings and that participants came to class prepared to take up the week's readings in a much more informed, focused and collaborative manner than had been the case in earlier versions of the course.

Issues that emerged outside class time (such as follow-ups to face-to-face meetings) and questions that students wanted others to answer or think about could be raised in the Readings online conference at the participants' convenience. We hoped this conference would also foster a sense of collaboration among the class members since they could have time to respond thoughtfully to each other's ideas and readings of texts at whatever length they choose and at times they met their individual schedules. We expected Summary conference and Readings conference to be mostly used by the class members, and this course structure seemed to meet the requirements for the new course format while allowing for high levels of out-of-class discussion.

Harasim et al. (1985) have suggested that the best indicator for the students of the importance of a course component is the weight it carries towards the final grade. To ensure the online component of the course was taken seriously by students, participation was worth 25% of their grade. Students were told that both the quality of the content of postings and the level of online interaction with other students would be part of the criteria for assigning participation marks. The remaining 75% of the grade was allocated to a symposium paper and publication-quality final essay on a topic of students' choice. Weighting the bulk of the course grade on individual student work was another way of promoting a learner-centered environment in which students were encouraged to focus on and share their own curiosities about modernist writers.

FINDINGS

Student participation in the online component of the course was tracked by using computer-generated usage statistics that summarized log-on times for each student throughout the course. In addition, the impressions of students were collected during and after the course through V-U pre- and post-use surveys and student course evaluations of the overall course, and the online component. Also, students posted reflections and comments about their impressions of the online conferences while the course was running.

Usage Statistics: Patterns of Student Participation in Online Discussions

The student and the instructor generated 154 messages in the online discussion as shown in Table 1. The large number of student postings in the Café conference (26 of 112 or 23%) reflects the fact that students used this conference early in the course as a test site (placing trial messages for each other and responding to others' messages). The Help

TABLE 1. Number of Messages in Each Conference by Students and Instructor

	Café	Help	Readings	Research	Summary	Subtotal
Students	26	14	15	14	43	112
Instructor	12	7	4	7	12	42
					Total	154

conference dealt primarily with technical problems (software configuration was the primary concern) and received 14% of the postings (21 of 154). As the course progressed, the bulk of the activity occurred in the Summary conference (55 of 154, or 36%), with much less activity in the Readings conference than had been anticipated (only 19 of 154 messages, or 12%). The Research conference gathered only 14% of postings (21 of 154), but most of these were postings from the middle to the end of the course as students became more focused on their term paper. Students did make use of the asynchronous capability of the online classroom by contributing postings at various times of the day and night: messages came in anytime between 7:00 a.m. and 10:00 p.m., as shown in Figure 1.

Students also logged on to the system seven days a week, and a definite pattern emerged in the breakdown of messages per day. Given that the course met on Monday afternoons, it is not surprising to see that the bulk of messages were posted on Sunday or Monday, in order to meet the deadline of posting summaries prior to the class meeting. Thirty-eight percent of postings came in on Sundays, and 17% on Mondays, for a total of 55% or 85 postings out of 154. A total of 69 postings (45%) came in on other days of the week, showing some discussion occurred between classes. However, less between-class discussion occurred than had been expected (Figure 2).

An analysis of the number of messages posted by each participant also revealed an interesting pattern, as shown in Figure 3. The mixed mode model, relying on both face-to-face and online teaching, apparently permitted some students to avoid using the online component. The four students all contributed to the online discussion, but to varying degrees; the least active contributed 15 messages (an average of 1.2 per week) and the most active had 40 messages (3.1 per week). Some students did little more than post the bare minimum required to submit their weekly summary. To put these numbers in perspective, we can contrast these findings with findings regarding students in courses that

FIGURE 1. Number of Messages by Hour of the Day

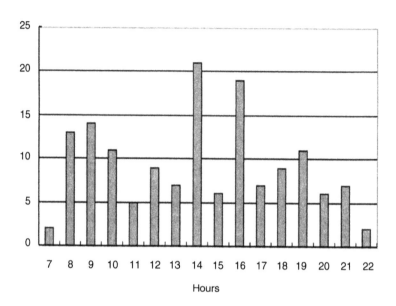

Hours

use only online communication (e.g., distance education online courses). Students in totally online courses tend to post more frequently, at an average of 10 messages per week per student (Wang & Teles, 1998).

Student Evaluation of the Online Experience

Initially, the graduate students were not enthusiastic about experimenting with online discussion. However, they soon started to participate more actively. The four students would not have classified themselves as being at the technological forefront, and most of them had some concerns about their level of computer literacy vis-à-vis the use of online discussion as an integral part of the course. An analysis of the surveys, course evaluations, and online postings completed by students revealed a mix of positive and negative reactions to the online experience. The benefits and problems reported by the students are discussed below.

Benefits of online group discussion. Participants saw learning how to use technology to enhance discussion as a benefit that went beyond the immediate purposes of the course. One student remarked, "I'm glad to

FIGURE 2. Number of Messages by Days of the Week

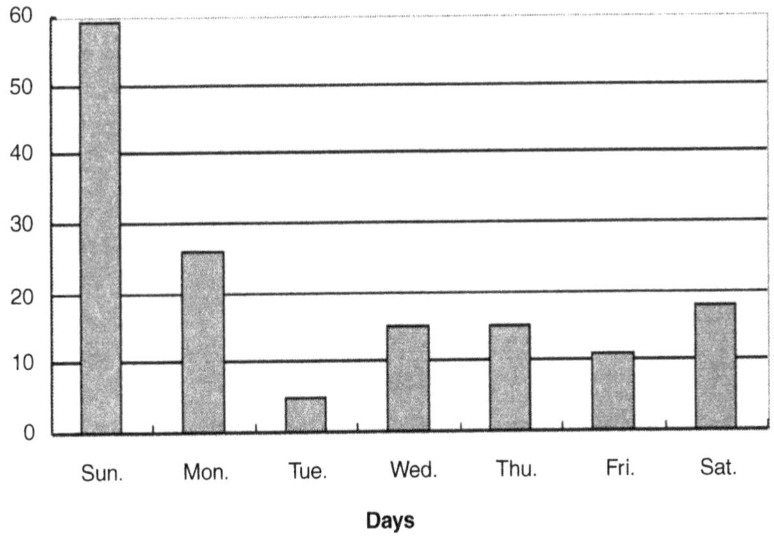

have had the exposure to the software and its possibilities (for myself and future teaching possibilities)."

There was appreciation for the pedagogical value of V-U. One student put it this way, "I really appreciated discussing my research on there and seeing everyone else's too. That's something that doesn't usually happen in a graduate class. Usually you only know what you're going to do, but I feel I know at least a little about everyone else's project . . . it gives more context." Students also felt that "In the context of the new two-hour courses, V-U is a valuable aid to increased communication." One important lesson we learned from these comments was that, by offering a forum in which students could discuss their individual research, and by actively encouraging them to share their research progress and strategies, we could further enhance student learning outcomes.

Another benefit reported by students was the concreteness of the final product: the students ended the course with a binder of written discussions, interpretations, and ideas that included a clear articulation of their own view on most of the issues raised in class, as well as the perspectives of four other people (the other students and the instructor) on the same issues. The students anticipated that the class discussions, frozen for future use, would be a valuable resource for future research and teaching in their field. Informal follow-ups with these students indi-

FIGURE 3. Number of Messages by Participants

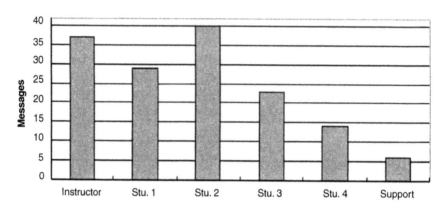

cated that this was the case; most reported that they had made more use of their course notes for this class than those from other courses.

Problems with online group discussions. Student difficulties arose in two main areas: technical problems and lack of experience with online group discussions. Students logging on to the class conferences from home experienced numerous problems. Memory limitations, incompatible modems, and other hardware-related problems plagued these students, which significantly downgraded the potential convenience of the asynchronous discussion. As one student noted, "What is the point of sending a message off into cyberspace when you're sitting next to the person you want to talk to?"

Modem access proved to be the single biggest technical difficulty faced by all class members. Because of the heavy demand on our university modem lines, students frequently had difficulty accessing the system. One student reported, "Access was an issue. Once I was ready to post on Friday, but couldn't get on until Sunday. Weekends are family time and I had to resend these messages, which often meant that my family's plans were interrupted because of the necessity of posting."

Students also identified a number of difficulties and dissatisfaction with the online group discussions themselves. The major problem was, in the words of one student, "It doesn't replace talking. Typing something is automatically more formal, and you miss the nuances of conversation, and the quick, digressive discussions that are often the most exciting part of classes." All the students agreed on this point, the implications of which will be discussed in a later section of this paper.

A second problem was students' differing perceptions of what the nature and length of postings should be. One student was frustrated by the fact that "I would (in an attempt to interact with others) raise issues, conversationally, in the summaries, that were never addressed." Another stated that, "Students should be strongly encouraged to be brief in their communications in any forum as time constraints on readers are extensive." And a third said, "I liked the potential of discussions. It was too bad they didn't really catch on until the end of the semester." The instructor's desire to have students carry on a substantial amount of the discussion online was not entirely fulfilled, most likely because of the differing perceptions of what they could or should do in this respect and also because of their difficulties in accessing the system.

A third problem was succinctly put in this student comment: "I had trouble with putting out statements in a vacuum." The lack of immediate personal feedback was felt by all the students. One suggested that "V-U would have been better with real-time discussion," while another suggested "that unless a V-U class time, when we would all be on at once, were set, real interaction was unlikely." Both comments suggest that students accustomed to a classroom situated learning style have difficulty envisioning asynchronous methods that are as effective and satisfying.

DISCUSSION

Given the experimental nature of this course design, it is important to investigate how well the course accomplished its objective. Four main administrative and pedagogical intentions for the course will be discussed: (a) quality of discussion; (b) effectiveness of asynchronicity; (c) impact of the learner-centered model; and (d) instructional workload.

Quality of Discussion

The mixed mode design was chosen to combine the immediacy of face-to-face discussion with the reflective potential of asynchronous online discussion, thus enhancing the quantity and quality of discussion in both modes. The extent to which these hopes were realized was mixed. Students and the instructor agreed that the online discussion did facilitate collaborative discussion and information sharing. However, several factors interfered with the online discussion emerging to the extent expected by the instructor. Technical barriers kept students from posting on a regular basis, and in a class of four the absence of any one individual was keenly felt. In addition, students who did post held different ideas of what was appropriate to post in terms of length and content. Some students posted long, conversation-like messages intended to prompt students to offer responses in kind. Other students were "put off" by lengthy messages. The lack of shared norms regarding appropriate postings in part led to a lack of responsiveness by others, which had a chilling effect on participation. Students were uncomfortable posting their thoughts into a "vacuum," with no guarantee of feedback.

Class size may have also impacted the quality of discussion online. Online conferences may need to be larger to generate active class discussions. However, the small number of students enabled the class to make the adjustments to the way they used V-U as difficulties arose, which may have been an important determinant in the success of the course. Whether a greater number of students would make more productive use of the online component of this course is hard to determine, but it is true that there would be more postings, and more students to respond to postings, which may result in greater dialogue.

The online discussion was also intended to enrich the face-to-face meetings. As discussed in a previous section, the in-class discussion was intentionally set up to start from where the online discussion left off, since classes always began with an overview of the posted reading summaries.

In contrast, the link between face-to-face meeting and the online conference was not explicitly supported in the course design, and did not emerge during the course. The online conferences were originally intended to create a space for students to raise issues and questions related to the face-to-face discussion as they came to mind during the week, in order to close the loop between the face-to-face and online conversations. However, not all issues raised face-to-face made their way online, even with the instructor's encouragement that students post questions they brought to her attention in order to get everyone's perspective.

Effectiveness of Asynchronicity

Students reported problems with the asynchronous nature of the online component of the course, largely because of a desire for more immediate feedback from the instructor and other students. Several students suggested the use of asynchronous online technologies (chatrooms). However, it is also important to point out that students did take advantage of the asynchronous nature of the online conference by posting at a variety of hours of the day and night, and all days of the week. Even in a class of four it may have been difficult to coordinate schedules to allow for synchronized discussion, and including the instructor in weekly chats would have defeated the purpose of cutting the face-to-face component down to two hours each week.

On the positive side, the implementation of a synchronous component might have been one way to allay student concerns about not having an immediate audience for their comments, and if done in conjunction with the asynchronous component, might have fostered greater comfort with and use of online discussion in general.

Slatin (1992) used a combination of synchronous and asynchronous technologies as well as face-to-face discussions to teach an upper-division course of 20th-century American poetry. His experience suggests that synchronous discussions can trigger significant online discussion throughout the week. One important finding Slatin offered is the importance of recognizing and framing online discussion as a legitimate model of teaching in its own right, rather than a necessary option used to meet budget restraints. Online interactive discussion, whether synchronous or asynchronous, "combines the informality and spontaneity of oral communication with the permanence of written discourse" and can create from this hybrid an intense and wide-ranging discussion of course topics (Slatin, 1992, p. 34). At least one student in this course clearly perceived the V-U mode as a less expensive stand-in for pedagogically preferred in-person teaching: "In my mind, 2-hour classes are in fact, half a 4-hour class and the V-U component does not in fact make up for the seminar time we would have exchanging ideas in person . . . With the shift to a more economically efficient course structure, I feel that the conditions under which knowledge is acquired and disseminated are increasingly chaotic." Clarifying the pedagogical rationale for online conferences to students may have helped to change this attitude.

Impact of Learner-Centered Model

Some of the dissatisfaction with the online component of the course seemed to stem from a discomfort with a learner-centered forum. The need for immediate feedback, especially from the instructor, could be part of a resistance to teaching models other than the dominant ones, such as lectures or classes led by an instructor whose responsibility is perceived as imparting a body of knowledge and stimulating discussion.

Students who have moved from undergraduate to graduate status seem to expect and even to prefer an enhanced vision of undergraduate courses. Often they want the familiar structure of professor leading the way augmented by intellectually more difficult and more stimulating material. Forums, which rely on student-initiated discussion, may be considered less valuable than forums that promise to offer the knowledge of an "expert." The growing appreciation of students for the specialized knowledge imparted by their colleagues in the discussion of their term projects represented a step toward the learner-centered goal of appreciating the expertise of peers and, by extension, their own expertise.

Latting (1994) analyzed the resistance of members of her graduate level social work class to asynchronous online conferencing. She found that resistance was related to complex social status issues within the classroom. Students split into "in-groups" and "out-groups" on the basis of their achievement motivation, level of computer access, and familiarity with Latting's teaching style. Once the class split into enthusiastic users and disgruntled non-users, no amount of face-to-face negotiation could stitch them back together again. Wegerif (1998) found familiar splits in a course on online teaching methods. These findings suggest caution in interpreting the meaning of resistance to online technology in the classroom. Although the English 803 class was too small to reveal clear cliques, the variation in the numbers of posting contributed by individual students and the differing ideas regarding appropriate length and content of postings suggest the potential volatility of even a very small online social system.

Instructor Workload

The final goal for this course was to provide a model that would help the instructor work within the limits of a reduced workload. This goal was not reached. The time needed to learn how to teach online was considerable. The very steep learning curve, even for an instructor who is relatively comfortable with computer technology, demands a large initial expenditure of time and energy. In the short term, we would have to say that the instructor puts in more effort than would be required in a similar course conducted entirely in the classroom. However, we believe that, once the initial stage passes, the instructor will reap the benefit of considerable time savings in future uses of V-U or other online teaching components.

CONCLUSIONS AND RECOMMENDATIONS

We felt that there was moderate success in using online group discussion for English 803. The online approach was very successful in providing a forum in which to place collective thoughts of the class about the texts studied in the course. The approach was also successful in creating a more collaborative atmosphere for students and the instructor. Students genuinely appeared to enjoy broadening their own specific interests by being able to see and discuss others' research. The potential problems, in terms of the loss of quality and content that were feared when the department embarked on its experimental graduate course format, did not materialize in this particular course.

In analyzing the student feedback, usage statistics, the nature of the postings to various conferences, and the instructor's experience, we came to see ways in which the design of the course might be improved. Some of these recommendations relate to overcoming technical difficulties, some involve a clarification of the pedagogical method for a mixed-mode course, and some have to do with challenging the students' preference for the prevailing pedagogical model.

Technical Difficulties

In the area of technical concerns, we would address three key points. First, we cannot assume that students are technologically adept, and therefore, it would be wise to schedule student training sessions in advance of the course so that early technical difficulties can be eliminated before the course begins. Second, there is a need for some sort of special modem access for courses so that the problems we encountered accessing the system do not prevent students from taking part in online learning. If institutions believe that technology is the answer to the problem of shrinking resources–that is, that computer learning can augment or replace classroom learning and provide a cost benefit advantage–then they must ensure that students have adequate access to computer facilities. Whether that access is on campus in the form of university supplied computer labs or, as is increasingly the case, from the students' own equipment through a modem, the university is ultimately responsible for ensuring that students can connect to the online environment with a minimum of difficulty. Third, the instructor's comfort level with online technology has a direct impact on the amount of time it takes to become familiar with teaching online. Initially, one can expect to spend more time, sometimes considerably more time, than in a more conventional course. However, once course development and instructional techniques that foster online collaboration are mastered, instructors will reap a time-savings dividend.

Clarifying Course Expectations

One way to enhance the quality and use of online discussion in this course might have been to model and insist that all questions raised off-line be posted online. A number of strategies might have structured this expectation into the course. Just as students were asked to present the reading summaries posted online to start in-class discussion, students could have also been assigned the task of summarizing the results of class discussion and posting the summary online. In addition, questions and issues raised with the instructor outside of class time could have been consistently referred to the online forum, and the importance of posting issues online could have been modeled by the instructor by having her take on the initial onus of posting issues raised with her. Once the expectation that all course discussion be placed online was established, students would be more likely to take on the responsibility of maintaining this policy.

Another way to encourage online discussion would have been to clarify expectations regarding the nature and length of postings in advance. For example, by stressing to students that their postings would not be judged as finished products but as contributions in an ongoing discourse, students would be encouraged to judge and modify their own submissions by looking at how much discussion was stimulated. The instructor also needed to be more explicit about what kinds of comments were to be posted in the Summary conference; indeed, "summary" was an ill-advised word choice because it suggested that the postings need only straight summaries of the readings rather than the more measured and engaged assessments of the material that she had hoped to see emerge.

Furthermore, it should have been made clearer at the beginning of the course that class members were expected to respond to postings in both a timely fashion—thereby lessening the sense of anxiety experienced by some when no one responded to their posting for several days— and in an intellectually engaged way. Had students who raised substantive issues been answered in kind by all members of the class, it is possible that more discussion would have ensued. Also, had their comments been answered quickly (within a day at most), the anxiety surrounding the sending of a message into the great void might well have been diminished.

The online component of the course accounted for 25% of the course grade; perhaps by increasing the percentage of grade given for online participation, and by more explicitly linking frequent and intellectual content of postings to the allocation of the grade, we might have been able to increase participation.

Finally, the use of synchronous online discussions might have sparked more use of online discussion in general. The instructor could set up number of regular real-time conferences, in addition to the face-to-face meetings and V-U conferences, to provide an area for real-time interaction among students and the instructor.

Broadening Pedagogical Horizons

The instructor has also learned about the pedagogical assumptions made about the "right" or "best" way to teach literature or any other discipline. Existing teaching paradigms need to be questioned–not necessarily with the agenda of replacing them with another model–but with the awareness that they, too, were once the challengers to an entrenched mode of teaching and learning. We do not advocate using computer learning as a replacement for face-to-face teaching; however, we believe that an online component can augment the current teaching models and can allow us to do a little more with a little less.

The growing use of online technology in higher education suggests another reason to use these methods with graduate students. As well as teaching our students the content of English Literature, we are also responsible for training them for future careers as college or university teachers. Familiarity with online technology helps to situate them favorably in the academic marketplace. Simply instructing them in how to use online databases, e-mail forums, or other Internet resources is not enough; we believe that our course's online component provided them with a model for how they might some day be asked to teach. By exposing them to the leading edge of online technology, we not only challenged the entrenched paradigm they were accustomed to, but we also challenged them as future teachers.

For many English instructors, computer technology means having access to e-mail/e-mail discussion groups, which enable us to keep in touch with colleagues around the world and with our students here at home. It also means being able to do some research via the Web (though we venture to suggest that no virtual encounter will replace the experience–both aesthetic and intellectual–of holding an unpublished essay written by T. S. Eliot). For the moment, the predominant teaching paradigm in English is the lecture/discussion format in which students and teachers place great emphasis on the immediacy of the give and take of ideas. Many English instructors point to the major limitations there have been until fairly recently in using online technology to recreate the lively interpersonal dynamics that constitute the heart and soul of the classroom learning situations for students and teachers alike. We think that online teaching to support classroom discussion has the potential to address this concern and that in so doing it will become an important part of both our teaching and technological repertoire. It provides a convenient form of information storage, retrieval, and access; at the same time, it allows students to collaborate in projects. Our experience convinces us that online learning has a place in the literature classroom, and we will continue to experiment with it to find the best ways to improve the use of online collaborative models.

REFERENCES

Bump, J. (1990). Radical changes in the class discussion using networked computers. *Computers and the Humanities, 24,* 49-65.

Harasim, L., Hiltz, R., Teles, L., & Turoff, M. (1995). *Learning networks: A field guide to teaching and learning online.* Cambridge, MA: MIT Press.

Hiltz, S.R. (1994). *The virtual classroom: Learning without limits via computer networks.* Norwood, NJ: Ablex.

Latting, J.K. (1994). Diffusion of computer-mediated communication in a graduate social work class: Lessons from "the class from hell." *Computers in Human Services, 10*(3), 21-45.

Moran, M.G. (1993, April). *The effect of budget cuts at the University of Georgia.* Paper presented at the Forty-Fourth Annual Meeting of the Conference on College Composition and Communication, San Diego, CA.

Slatin, J.M. (1992). Is there a class in this text? Creating knowledge in the electronic classroom. In E. Barrett (Ed.), *Sociomedia: Multimedia, hypermedia, and the social construction of knowledge* (pp. 27-52). Cambridge, MA: MIT Press.

Wang, X., & Teles, L. (1998, October). *Online collaboration and the role of the instructor in two university credit courses.* Paper presented at the International Conference of Computers in Education, Beijing, China.

Wegerif, R. (1998). The social dimension of asynchronous learning. *Journal of Asynchronous Learning Networks, 2*(1). Retrieved July 16, 1999 from the World Wide Web: *http://www.aln.org/alnweb/journal/jaln_vol2issue1.htm*

Christine Mayer
Dale Musser
Herbert Remidez

Description of a Web-Driven, Problem-Based Learning Environment and Study of the Efficacy of Implementation in Educational Leader Preparation

SUMMARY. A Web-driven problem-based learning environment and instructional system was conceived and developed to study the marriage of the problem-based learning instructional method and Web technologies for instructional delivery of educational administration content material. The project described herein was undertaken to examine the efficacy of implementing this new mode of instruction in graduate courses in educational leadership. The ultimate goal of this line of research is to enhance the development of applications of Web technologies to support problem-based learning and improve the efficiency and

CHRISTINE MAYER is Professor, University of Missouri-Columbia, Center for Technology Innovations in Education, 111 London Hall, Columbia, MO 65211 (E-mail: Mayer@coe.missouri.edu).
DALE MUSSER is Assistant Professor, University of Missouri-Columbia, School of Information Science and Learning Technology, 111 London Hall, Columbia, MO 65211 (E-mail: MusserDa@coe.missouri.edu).
HERBERT REMIDEZ is Doctoral Student, University of Missouri-Columbia, School of Information Science and Learning Technology, 111 London Hall, Columbia, MO 65211 (E-mail: RemidezH@coe.missouri.edu).

[Haworth co-indexing entry note]: "Description of a Web-Driven, Problem-Based Learning Environment and Study of the Efficacy of Implementation in Educational Leader Preparation." Mayer, Christine, Dale Musser, and Herbert Remidez. Co-published simultaneously in *Computers in the Schools* (The Haworth Press, Inc.) Vol. 18, No. 1, 2001, pp. 249-265; and: *The Web in Higher Education: Assessing the Impact and Fulfilling the Potential* (ed: Cleborne D. Maddux, and D. LaMont Johnson) The Haworth Press, Inc., 2001, pp. 249-265. Single or multiple copies of this article are available for a fee from The Haworth Document Delivery Service [1-800-342-9678, 9:00 a.m. - 5:00 p.m. (EST). E-mail address: getinfo@haworthpressinc.com].

249

efficacy of this instructional form in practice across higher education settings. This article describes the prototype software, the rationale and theoretical framework supporting its development, the process and results of research conducted during production and beta-testing, and the educational significance of the project. *[Article copies available for a fee from The Haworth Document Delivery Service: 1-800-342-9678. E-mail address: <getinfo@haworthpressinc.com> Website: <http://www.HaworthPress.com>*

KEYWORDS. Web-based instruction, problem-based learning, educational administration, software development, higher education, Web technologies, school leader preparation, digital learning environments

Since the 1950s the training of educational leaders at colleges and universities has included "in-basket" exercises and simulations, which defined administrative work as the problems that find the administrator, rather than emphasizing the administrator's capacity to engage in reflective problem finding. Problems in educational leadership, however, are not that clear-cut and are often ill structured; problems are typically not distinctly defined, involve several simultaneous conceptual structures, and are irregular across cases. Like many professional domains, educational leadership is a domain where, at the advanced level, there are no clear-cut right or wrong answers and an understanding of the domain requires the simultaneous understanding of often-conflicting viewpoints. The problem-based learning approach was first broadly applied to educational leadership to correct flaws of the in-basket approach (Bridges & Hallinger, 1992). Although agreement exists on the merits of problem-based learning, the success of this method of instruction depends upon many variables whose handling is challenging, even for the most dedicated and experienced instructor.

Applications of World Wide Web technologies have been designed to support, enrich, and expand learning and to improve the efficiency, efficacy, and authenticity of instruction in higher education. The Web has quickly emerged as a powerful, global, interactive, and dynamic means for teaching and learning. The literature abounds with examples of innovative instructors using the Web to deliver, enhance, and expand instruction. What has not been clearly articulated, however, is what happens when problem-based learning is delivered by way of a Web-based learning environment.

A Web-driven problem-based learning environment and instructional system was conceived by the University Council for Educational Administration (UCEA), a consortium of 56 research universities having doctoral programs in educational administration. The prototype software was then developed by the University of Missouri-Columbia Center for Technology Innovations in Education to study the marriage of the problem-based learning instructional method and Web technologies for instructional delivery of educational administration content material. While the project described herein was undertaken to examine the efficacy of implementing this new mode of instruction in graduate courses in educational leadership, the ultimate goal of this line of research is to enhance the development of applications of Web technologies to support problem-based learning and improve the efficiency and efficacy of this instructional form in practice across higher education settings.

DESCRIPTION OF THE PROTOTYPE SOFTWARE

The Information Environment for School Leader Preparation (IESLP; pronounced "I-Slip") (http://ieslp.coe.missouri.edu) is a Web-driven problem-based instructional system and information environment that uses the tools of technology to place educational leaders in the virtual halls, classrooms, and boardrooms of actual schools, providing a safe opportunity for learners to explore real situations and develop reflective expertise. It draws practitioners and would-be educational leaders into ways of thinking that incorporate the use of technological resources, tools, information, theory, and research. It creates a demand to make reflective, information-based decisions and engage in collegial problem finding and intervention.

With the problem-based learning approach, learners collaborate to study the facets of a real-world problem as they strive to create viable solutions. IESLP and problem-based learning are grounded in the same pedagogical approach. IESLP, however, fosters the use of Web and information technologies to provide students with opportunities to build skill in identifying problems and opportunities; generating proactive solutions; and encouraging collegial approaches to intervention and the acquisition of knowledge, skills, and dispositions appropriate for leadership in contemporary educational organizations. The IESLP approach challenges learners to use technological resources to solve problems and demonstrate learning through varied authentic activities. The system was designed with the intention of changing the way those who prepare educational leaders think about knowledge, information, technology, research, the practice of educational administration, and ultimately, about modifying the behaviors of researchers, instructors, and the practitioners of educational leadership.

IESLP is not a computer simulation, but computing technology is an integral part of IESLP. Instead of acting on problem exercises in a simulated computer environment, IESLP exercises are worked on by people in face-to-face groupings, using technology as they will in their actual work. That is, students use technological tools to retrieve information and data, analyze data, communicate, and produce products. Unlike a simulation, in IESLP this is done in the context of human work groups, subject to the uncertainties and limitations of those groups, just as teams of administrators do in real educational settings.

IESLP, therefore, is much more than a traditional simulation could be. It is a comprehensive information learning environment that brings to learners and instructors the genuine complexity of contemporary schools. While older style simulations based on in-basket exercises tended to define school administration in terms of coping with problems that find administrators, the IESLP system is based on another idea: that the most critical skills administrators can develop are those having to do with problem identification, problem framing, problem intervention, and problem prevention (Hallinger, Leithwood, & Murphy, 1993; Leithwood & Stager, 1989).

Four essential components constitute the strength and uniqueness of the IESLP software: (a) problem exercises, (b) community and school environments, (c) communication features, and (d) tools and resources.

Problem Exercises

IESLP learning begins with authentic, ill-structured problems of professional practice. The exercises address a broad range of issues surrounding K-16 education with a particular K-12 emphasis. Unlike in-basket approaches, in which problems are given and highly constrained, IESLP problem exercises vary along a continuum from virtually unconstrained problem identification to highly constrained problems similar to in-basket exercises. The IESLP system is designed to socialize leaders to analyze and use information from a variety of sources, including research, community and school data, and the acquired wisdom of experts and colleagues in the resolution of problems. Exercises can be described as falling on a continuum framed by "problem finding" to "problem presented." In problem-finding exercises, learners are asked to define and shape the problem/opportunity with little direction. Problem-finding exercises address the belief that professional problem identification and framing are among the most critical skills for successful school leadership. Thus, these problem exercises take the form of very general and ill-structured charges. Assignments to learners are unconstrained, and the problem as well as the solution is to be discovered. As a result, the approaches, problem definitions, decisions about interventions, and work products can vary a great deal from one learner work group to another. In contrast, problem-presented exercises provide learners with more information, more constraint, and create rather specific expectations about products required of individuals and learner groups. Problem-presented exercises may place time limitations, process requirements, product specifications, and other constraints on the exercise. The following criteria further distinguish these two problem types:

1. Interface–the extent to which the exercise relies on the background materials, the IESLP community and school environments, and the professional research base;
2. Constraint–the extent to which the exercise is limited by instructions (is the problem to be found or is it given), and;
3. Consequence–the extent to which earlier actions and decisions of the learner group constrain succeeding choices.

The catalyst is the starting point for a particular exercise. It is an ill-structured problem, issue, or situation that will be the opening focus of individual and group activity and exploration. The catalyst can take a variety of shapes and forms. Bridges and Hallinger (1992) talk about the catalyst this way: "Each project is structured around a high-impact problem that the administrator is apt to face in the future. A high-impact problem is one that has the potential to affect large numbers of people for an extended period of time. Some of these problems are highly structured, while others are complex, messy, and ill-defined" (p. 21).

Community and School Environments

IESLP's community and school environments create an authentic backdrop in front of which a wide variety of learning activities can take place. IESLP provides users with access to an extended set of data from actual community and school settings that serve as the setting for problem/opportunity discovery, examination of relevant research and best practice knowledge, and group negotiation of decisions about appropriate interventions. The information provided in the community and school environments is comprehensive and provides a context in which students can engage in problems of practice. The environments are community and school Web sites constructed with authentic information collected from actual schools and their surrounding communities, including community demographics, district information, school characteristics, and information on facilities, budget, students, parents, and teachers. The data in the environments are real, but modified to protect identities. The IESLP community and school environments vary by educational level and community type. Data contained in the first environment included in the IESLP system were collected in a rural Oklahoma public school district. Future environments currently under development will include the city of Houston and the Houston Independent School District as the urban environment and a yet-to-be-named suburban public school district and the community it is situated in as the suburban environment.

Communication Features

The IESLP system includes built-in communication features that allow users to work closely with members of their IESLP work groups, even though they might be separated by distance. Much of the work students will undertake while using IESLP will be done in the context of groups. For numerous reasons, however, electronic communication and correspondence are often necessary. The IESLP communications system includes features that enable users to send and receive messages via message boards and to "chat" or talk one-on-one with people across the Internet using real-time text. The message boards provide a means for asynchronous communication within a class or among all IESLP users. These features can also act as the means for community discussions and debates. The system enables instructors to send out tasks and monitor student progress, and enables students to submit the products of their work to their instructor via the IESLP system.

Tools and Resources

IESLP includes links to the appropriate analytical tools and research in education and the social sciences, and fosters the routine and intelligent use of both. The information environment encourages learning and skill building responsive to the genuine problems and opportunities found in schools. Consistent with the notion of providing rich, authentic learning experiences that include skill learning objectives, IESLP exercises incorporate information management, data analysis, decision making, reporting, problem solving, and presentation. Many of the tools required to complete tasks are available on the Web, and a number of them at the Planet Innovation Web site (*http://planet.rtec.org/*). Also developed at the University of Missouri-Columbia Center for Technology Innovations in Education, Planet Innovation tools support decision makers as they plan, implement, and evaluate programs, particularly K-12 technology planning. To facilitate the decision-making process, Planet Innovation has an on-demand Web environment through which individuals can choose Web solutions based on their needs and, if desired, form groups to work in a distributed environment. The Planet Innovation tools assist the planning and decision-making process by supporting communication and informed choices.

THEORETICAL FRAMEWORK

In 1993 the American Psychological Association released a report entitled, "Learner-Centered Psychological Principles: A Framework for School Redesign and Reform." According to this report, an effective curriculum includes genuine problems and learner performance appraisals that are congruous to real-life situations. About the same time, the California Commission on Teacher Credentialing (1993) issued a report identifying the need to reconstruct the professional preparation of educational administrators so that it is more closely tied to the complex problems facing practitioners. In contrast to traditional instruction, new modes of authentic instruction are needed in which instruction normally occurs within small discussion groups of learners that are facilitated by an instructor serving as the mentor (Aspy, Aspy, & Quimby, 1993; Bridges & Hallinger, 1992). Problem-based learning is a learner-driven pedagogical approach for posing significant problems of practice in the context of real-world situations while providing resources, guidance, and instruction to learners as they build content knowledge and problem-solving skills, and strive to devise viable solutions or interventions (Aspy, Aspy, & Quimby, 1993; Bridges & Hallinger, 1992; Mayo, Donnelly, Nash, & Schwartz, 1993).

The goal in designing the IESLP software was to foster more effective methods for preparing educational leaders. In doing so, we sought to facilitate more authentic avenues for teaching and learning school leadership and to encourage the use of information technology in the practice of school leadership. We also sought to introduce into program curricula the knowledge, skills, and values that are more directly related to successful school leadership (Starratt, 1993). Three assumptions undergirded the development of IESLP:

1. One of the most essential skills for school leaders is aggressive problem/opportunity identification (Leithwood & Hallinger, 1993; Leithwood & Stager, 1989).
2. Schools will be most successful when professional staff members work together under an ethos of collegiality.
3. Professional knowledge (including that of the school leader) is partly transferable, partly experiential, and partly intuitive, artful, and morally reflective in context (Schön, 1987; Short & Rinehart, 1993).

The developers of the IESLP concept visualized school leader preparation that meets these assumptions.

IESLP's design embodies a theme of reflective practice and is grounded in contemporary learning theory. A single learning theory is not the answer to all instructional situations. Nor have we yet discovered all there is to know about learning. As a consequence, educational practitioners can do no more than make informed judgments about what theories have the most to offer in a particular instructional situation. The approach taken in the development of the IESLP instructional approach was not intended to be all-inclusive, but to review prominent learning theories and utilize those that have relevance, merit, and generalizability in educational administration, and more broadly, in higher education.

The IESLP system embraces multiple learning theories that have proved effective in instruction, all of which are complementary to Web-driven problem-based learning. Despite differences among theories, they share assumptions. First, they refer to learning as a persisting change in human performance or performance potential. That is, learners are capable of actions they could not perform before learning occurred and this is true whether they actually have an opportunity to exhibit the newly acquired performance. As evident in the IESLP problem exercises, this approach challenges learners to demonstrate learning through varied authentic problems. Second, to be considered learning, a change in performance must come about as a result of the learner's interaction with the environment. The selected theories are well integrated with one another and the strengths of each have been embedded in the IESLP approach. A brief description of how each contributes to the IESLP approach is provided below.

Schema theory looks at the interconnected nature of how information is organized in the human mind. Humans link what is heard, seen, touched, and tasted with what is already known. The better connected the organizational network in the long-term memory, the better and faster one can assess information and make sound decisions (Arbib, 1989). A schema is "a data structure for representing the generic concepts stored in memory" (Rumelhart, 1980, p. 34). Schemata are packets of knowledge, and schema theory is a theory of how these packets are represented and how that representation facilitates the use of the knowledge in particular ways. In developing the IESLP approach, careful consideration was given to the question, How might traditional instruction be changed to encourage the development of schema? Schemata acquisition is encouraged by exposure to examples of the schema. Pairing examples and matched non-examples supports schema refinement. The IESLP approach was designed to encourage schema formation and refinement. One way to encourage schema formation in instruction is through small group work. Schema formation and refinement occur when group members ask one another questions and explain why they are solving something in a certain way. Schema development occurs in IESLP when small groups work together toward resolution of the problem exercises.

Generative learning theory asserts that people tend to generate perceptions and meanings that are consistent with their prior learning. The learner is an active participant in the process and constructs meaning based on prior knowledge. Learning is a function of the abstract, distinctive, and concrete associations the learner generates between prior experiences, as they are stored in memory, and incoming stimuli (Duffy & Jonassen, 1992). Learning with understanding, then, is a process of generating semantic and distinctive idiosyncratic associations between stimuli and stored information. The effects of instruction to generate transfer and relationships depend on the learner's general abilities and specific relevant experience and information-processing strategies.

Constructivism also emphasizes learning in context. The knowledge that learners can usefully deploy should be developed in the context of meaningful activity that allows learners to build upon what is already understood. Learning conditions should include complex learning environments that incorporate authentic activity, provide for social negotiation as an integral part of learning, juxtapose instructional content and include access to multiple modes of representation, nurture reflexivity, and emphasize learner-centered instruction (Brooks & Brooks, 1993). The instructional approach taken by IESLP incorporates many of the principles identified with constructivism. Ill-defined situations that are taken on by a work group of three to four learners provide the authentic environment for wrestling with and discerning significant problems and devising intervention plans. Whole class sessions to critique intervention strategies emphasize the social negotiation aspect of constructivism. Central to IESLP is the emphasis on the learner taking responsibility and taking charge of the situation. The instruction is learner-centered.

Cognitive flexibility theory is an extension of constructivism that is more specifically responsive to advanced learning in ill-structured domains. Cognitive flexibility theory emphasizes presentation of learning experiences in authentic, complex, and ill-structured contexts. The design of instruction utilizing the cognitive flexibility approach must provide for multiple passes through instructional material and the presentation of multiple perspectives on issues. In addition, the application of a concept under study should be shown in the diverse situations in which it might actually appear. The lesson design should provide for learner reflection. The design of instruction utilizing the cognitive flexibility approach enables the learner to structure, integrate, and interconnect new ideas with previous ones (Spiro, Feltovich, Jacobson, & Coulson, 1992). Multiplicity of information can, perhaps, confound an issue, but in real-life problems are seldom straightforward. The effective resolution of problems requires reflection on the multiple issues, perspectives, and information at hand. The IESLP approach demonstrates to the learner the true complexity of solving problems and the resources that can shed more light on the problem-solving process. Learner reflection is encouraged as new information is obtained and is integrated with previous information.

The work of John Keller involving motivational theory has important implications and applications for instruction. An understanding of how to arouse and maintain student interest applies to both the designers of Web-driven problem-based learning environments like IESLP and to IESLP instructors and learners, who are also educational practitioners. Central to this work are four major dimensions of motivation: (a) interest, which refers to whether the learner's curiosity is aroused and whether this arousal is sustained appropriately over time; (b) relevance, which refers to whether the learner perceives the instruction to satisfy personal needs or to help achieve personal goals; (c) expectancy, which refers to the learner's perceived likelihood of success and the extent to which he or she perceives success as being under his or her control; and (d) satisfaction, which refers to the learner's intrinsic motivations and his or her reactions to extrinsic rewards (Keller, 1983).

The IESLP project draws on four main elements of adult learning theory: (a) self-direction, (b) personal experiences used as resources, (c) immediate application, and (d) learning readiness tied to the roles they play in the workplace (Brookfield, 1986).

Meaningful reception learning theory asserts that learning is not something that resides "in the text" and outside of the learner. Textual materials, like anything else learners might experience, are only to be considered potentially meaningful. Meaning occurs when learners actively interpret their experience using certain internal, cognitive operations (Ausubel, Novak, & Hanesian, 1978). To account for these cognitive operations and how they interact with experience to give rise to learning, the theory of meaningful reception learning was proposed. Meaningful learning refers to the process of relating potentially meaningful information to what the learner already knows in a nonarbitrary and substantive way (Ausubel, 1963). The driving force behind the IESLP approach is to make the learning experience meaningful. Exercises focus on skill building in problem finding, framing, and identification. Skill-building processes emphasize the integration of external resources with the internal, cognitive operations of the learner. Learners are provided the means to access information and resources and are then provided the opportunity and time to assimilate this information in meaningful ways. Small group and large group work assist the learner in making sense of the situation and information. The active participation of the learner throughout the IESLP learning experience facilitates the internal processing and meaningfulness of the learning.

Metacognitive theory has the greatest impact on the design of current instructional studies (Osman & Hannafin, 1992). This theoretical approach has highlighted the importance of strategy maintenance and transfer and has investigated two forms of training: informed training and self-control training. The IESLP approach provides for both types of training through its problem exercises and supporting tools and resources. Learners become much more successful at determining appropriate strategies to use in problem-solving situations, and at monitoring actions and outcomes along the way. In *informed training*, learners are given the rationale of the strategy to be learned and are helped to see the direct relationship between the strategy use and subsequent increased learning. The use of informed training has resulted in successful maintenance of learning strategy in learners (Paris, Newman, & McVey,

1982). In *self-control training*, learners are instructed in executive control functions as well as specific strategy. Executive control functions include planning, checking, monitoring, and overseeing the activity or activities induced. The guiding principles of self-control training are twofold: (a) to teach learners how to learn rather than only what to learn; and (b) to teach learners to spontaneously plan, check, and monitor themselves in their learning, performance, and problem solving. The advantage of self-control training lies in the learners' maintenance and generalization of learned strategies (Osman & Hannafin, 1992). Informed training differs from self-control training in the following manner. The informed training approach focuses on providing the learners with a clear rationale of the strategy to be trained and on the direct relationship between strategy use and its beneficial effects on learning. Self-control training focuses on direct instruction of general executive skills, such as planning, checking, and monitoring, as well as on help with overseeing and coordinating the activity (Brown, Bransford, Ferrara, & Campione, 1983).

With the advent of powerful new technologies easily accessible by the masses, Siegel and Kirkley (1997) describe the need for a new teaching and learning paradigm, which they call "digital learning environments." This type of learning environment would provide safe but authentic settings for teaching and learning in which students have the opportunity and guidance to learn from their mistakes while employing problem-solving strategies in real-world contexts (Shank, 1994). The Web provides an open, dynamic information architecture to host and deliver new learning environments (Siegel & Sousa, 1994). The assumption underlying this project was that delivery of problem-based learning by way of an electronic learning environment would allow learners to be challenged to use technological resources to solve authentic problems of practice and demonstrate learning through varied authentic activities.

Process of Inquiry

As a beginning point in studying the efficiency and efficacy of implementing Web-driven problem-based learning environments, the software prototype was built and a study was conducted of the factors that contribute to instructors' decisions regarding adoption, including the benefits and barriers to implementation. The research design was grounded in the qualitative tradition based on the theoretical assumptions underpinning qualitative research. These assumptions are that "meaning and process are crucial in understanding human behavior, that descriptive data are imperative and must come from the participants' perspective, and that analysis is best done inductively" (Bogdan & Biklen, 1998, p. 50).

Qualitative research data from typical end users of IESLP (faculty and students in educational leadership programs) were collected and triangulated by the following means: questionnaires, interviews, informal meetings, demonstrations, online chat sessions, e-mail communications, user tracking scripts, learner artifacts, and message boards. Data were coded and analyzed using the methods for developing grounded theory as espoused by Strauss and Corbin (1998).

SUMMARY OF FINDINGS

Research done during the development of the prototype software was instrumental in informing both the ongoing development process as well as contributing to the output of a successful system prototype for others in higher education to emulate. Studies conducted of typical end users ($n = 10$ instructors, 100 students) show that instructors and students must undergo a significant change in teaching and learning paradigm and be fully oriented to the Web-driven problem-based learning environment before their engagement is successful. For optimal use of IESLP, research has shown that students and instructors must commit to its learning methodology and become familiar with the system and facile in its use. Consequently, when used, IESLP should be the focal instructional approach.

Instructors can build syllabi using IESLP to address all of the learning objectives they have identified for a given course. Ideally, once instructors and students have oriented to IESLP, it can provide the starting point for many courses in preparation programs for educational leaders. IESLP was found to be a flexible and comprehensive instructional system that can be used to teach regular university courses in school leadership and administration, as well as to provide continuing education opportunities for practicing administrators. Results also indicated that this instructional approach facilitates the integration of the various subdisciplines that now fragment the teaching and learning of school administration, and enables educational administration professors to collaborate in the use of problem-based learning approaches and instructional styles suited to adult learners. The IESLP problem exercises and information environments can be used to deliver administration, finance, law, organizational theory, instructional supervision, learning theory, and other content, either through traditionally focused courses sorted by these subdisciplines, or through an integrated sequence of cross-disciplinary courses.

Successful IESLP engagement requires that both instructors and students accept the blurring of traditional roles, allowing for the instructor to provide an unprescribed amount of guidance and serve as a mentor while the students facilitate and manage their own learning experience. Further, both instructors and students must attain a level of comfort with technology and proficiency with using a Web browser that will facilitate effective use of the software. Once instructors and students are fully oriented, however, this teaching and learning construct closely parallels the limitations, stresses, and processes of work in the real world in a safe but authentic environment. Our work suggests that electronic learning environments can bridge the gap between content-centered instruction and cooperative, learner-driven, problem-centered preparation of future educational leaders to deal with all types of practical situations in which they might eventually find themselves, using information technology as a resource.

By the time learners finished the IESLP program, they had developed their own informed views of learning and administrative approaches. Learners were ready to take a stand on the merits of particular administrative theories and approaches as they might be applied to various educational and instructional problems. Learners felt in a position to identify gaps in theory and administrative practice, and to suggest directions for future research. In essence, learners ultimately measure the effectiveness of IESLP as they become reflective practitioners.

Research results suggest that the marriage of Web-based learning environments and problem-based instruction can be effective in providing students access to a multitude of collaboration, productivity, communication, and knowledge creation tools that enrich the learning experience. For instructors, flexible electronic learning environments can provide management tools that allow for success in mentoring and guiding rich collaborative learning experiences for use in traditional classroom or distance learning settings. Respondents agreed that, although the novel teaching and learning paradigm was ultimately effective, the challenges that exist in altering teaching pedagogy and learning paradigms present a roadblock to implementing this approach.

Educational Significance

Our study found that Web-driven problem-based learning environments can provide an authentic approach to building skills in identifying problems and opportunities, generating proactive solutions, and encouraging collegial approaches to intervention, while fostering the acquisition of knowledge, skills, and dispositions appropriate for leadership in contemporary educational organizations. Research results concluded that this teaching and learning construct stimulates a revolutionary departure from predominant patterns of administrator preparation using authentic avenues for teaching and learning school leadership, and encourages the use of information technology in the practice of school leadership. Thinking and acting in the real and imperfect environments provided by this type of electronic learning environment closely parallels the limitations, stresses, and processes of work in the real-world and prepares future educational leaders to deal with all types of situations in which they might eventually find themselves.

The assumptions and needs underlying the development of this type of teaching and learning construct are not specific to educational administration, but are common to all disciplines and the careers with which they are linked. This type of electronic learning environment can be designed and created to transform the preparation of any type of professional into an experience that teaches critical discipline-specific content knowledge, but also and perhaps more importantly, provides learner-driven opportunities to work with real problems of practice in a safe but authentic environment before the professional enters the workplace. The system encourages collaboration among instructors and learners and can be used for traditional classroom or distributed learning. Finally, the system encourages learners to think about problems and solutions in unique and informed ways, and to use information technology as a resource.

REFERENCES

American Psychological Association. (1993). *Learner-centered psychological principles: A framework for school redesign and reform.* Washington, DC: Spielberger, C. D., Clark, L. A., Feshbach, N. D., Kintsch, W., Lambe, N. M., McCombs, B. L., Rosenfield, S. A., Tenopyr, M., & Weinstein, C. E.

Arbib, M. A. (1989). *The metaphorical brain 2: Neural networks and beyond.* New York: Wiley-Interscience.

Aspy, D. N., Aspy, C. B., & Quimby, P. M. (1993). What doctors can teach teachers about problem-based learning. *Educational Leadership, 50*(7), 22-24.

Ausubel, D. P. (1963). *The psychology of meaningful verbal learning.* New York: Grune & Stratton.

Ausubel, D. P., Novak, J. D., & Hanesian, H. (1978). *Educational psychology: A cognitive view* (2nd ed.). New York: Holt, Rinehart & Winston.

Birch, L. (1993). *Preparation, induction, and professional growth of school administrators.* Sacramento, CA: California Commission on Teacher Credentialing.

Bogdan, R. C., & Biklen, S. K. (1998). *Qualitative research in education: An introduction to theory and methods* (3rd ed.). Boston, MA: Allyn & Bacon.

Bridges, E. M., & Hallinger, P. (1992). *Problem-based learning for administrators.* Eugene, OR: ERIC Clearinghouse on Educational Management.

Brookfield, Stephen D. (1986). *Understanding and facilitating adult learning.* San Francisco: Jossey-Bass.

Brooks, J. G., & Brooks, M. G. (1993). *In search of understanding: The case for constructivist classrooms.* Alexandria, VA: Association for the Supervision and Curriculum Development.

Brown, A. L., Bransford, J. D., Ferrara, R. A., & Campione, J. C. (1983). Learning, remembering and understanding. In W. Damon (Ed.), *Handbook of child psychology,* 4th ed. (pp. 77-166). New York: Wiley & Sons.

Duffy, T., & Jonassen, D. (Eds.). (1992). Constructivism and the technology of instruction: A conversation. In T. M. Duffy & D. H. Jonassen (Eds.), *Technology and the design of generative learning environments* (pp. 77-89). Hillsdale, NJ: Erlbaum.

Hallinger, P., Leithwood, K. A., & Murphy, J. (Eds.) (1993). *Cognitive perspectives on educational leadership.* New York, NY: Teachers College Press.

Keller, J. M. (1983). Motivational design of instruction. In C. M. Reigeluth (Ed.), *Instructional design theories and models: An overview of their current status.* Hillsdale, NJ: Erlbaum.

Leithwood, K. A., & Hallinger, P. (1993). Cognitive perspectives on educational administration: An introduction. *Educational Administration Quarterly, 29*(3), 296-301.

Leithwood, K. A., & Stager, M. (1989). Expertise in principals' problem solving. *Educational Administration Quarterly, 25*(2), 126-161.

Mayo, P., Donnelly, M. B., Nash, P. P., & Schwartz, R. W. (1993). Student perceptions of tutor effectiveness in problem based surgery clerkship. *Teaching and Learning in Medicine, 5*(4), 227-233.

Osman, M. E., & Hannafin, M. J. (1992). Metacognition research and theory: Analysis and implications for instructional design. *Educational Technology Research and Development, 40*(2), 83-99.

Paris, S. G., Newman, R. S., & McVey, K. A. (1982). Learning the functional significance of mnemonic actions: A microgenetic study of strategy acquisition. *Journal of Experimental Child Psychology, 34*, 490-509.

Rumelhart, D. E. (1980). Schemata: The building blocks of cognition. In R. J. Spiro, B. Bruce, & R. W. Brewer (Eds.), *Theoretical issues in reading comprehension* (pp. 33-58). Hillsdale, NJ: Erlbaum.

Schön, D. A. (1987). *Educating the reflective practitioner.* San Francisco, CA: Jossey Bass.

Shank, R. C. (1994). Why hitchhikers on the information highway are going to have to wait a long time for a ride. *The Aspen Institute Quarterly, 6*(2), 28-58.

Short, P. M., & Rinehart, J. S. (1993). Reflections as a means of developing expertise. *Educational Administration Quarterly, 29*(4), 501-521.

Siegel, M. A., & Kirkley, S. (1997). Moving toward the digital learning environment: The future of Web-based instruction. In B. H. Khan (Ed.), *Web-based instruction* (pp. 263-270). Englewood Cliffs, NJ: Educational Technology Publications.

Siegel, M. A., & Sousa, G. A. (1994). Inventing the virtual textbook: Changing the nature of schooling. *Educational Technology, 34*(7), 49-54.

Spiro, R. J., Feltovich, P. J., Jacobson, M. J., & Coulson, R. L. (1992). Cognitive flexibility, constructivism, and hypertext: Random access instruction for advanced knowledge acquisition in ill-structured domains. In T. M. Duffy & D. H. Jonassen (Eds.), *Constructivism and the technology of instruction: A conversation* (pp. 57-75). Hillsdale, NJ: Erlbaum.

Starratt, R. J. (1993). *The drama of leadership.* Washington, DC: The Falmer Press.

Strauss, A., & Corbin, J. (1998). *Basics of qualitative research: Techniques and procedures for developing grounded theory* (2nd ed.). Thousand Oaks, CA: Sage Publications.

Index

A *Nation at Risk*, 5
ACEI. *See* Association for
    Childhood Education
    International (ACEI)
Adler, M.J., 18
After-School Online Discussions,
    112
Aims, defined, 51
Alcott, B., 24-25,26
American Automobile Association, 4
American Literature site, 28-29
Analytical reading, 19-20
Anger
    at government-related activities,
      6-7
    national epidemic of, 5
Artifact(ies), technological, 2
Ashton, S., 231
Asking the Right Questions, 19
Association for Childhood Education
    International (ACEI), 10
Asynchronicity, of online classroom
    interaction to enhance
    graduate instruction in
    English Literature,
    effectiveness of, 242-243
Attitude(s), in cognitive flexibility
    hypertext for developing
    sexual harassment cases,
    224-225,225f
Aviv, R., 80

Bandura, A., 99
Barab, S.A., 107,108,110,123
Barnard, J., 88
Beauvis, K., 224,226

Berman, P., 131-132
Binker, 24
BlackBoard, 43
Bonk, C.J., 27-28,189
Boud, D., 84
Bridges, E.M., 253
Brown, J.S., 109,110
Browne, M.N., 19
Bureau of Alcohol, Tobacco, and
    Firearms, anger directed at, 6

California Commission on Teacher
    Credentialing, 255
Capitalism, laissez-faire, vs.
    education, 11
Carey, L., 44
Case quality, 197,199t
Case relevance, 197-198,199t
Case-based learning
    historical background of,
      191-192
    in pre-service teacher training,
      191-211
      described, 192-193
      future directions in, 209-210
      pedagogical and technology rec-
        ommendations in, 208-209
      study of, 193-197,194f
        case evaluations in, 196-197
        case quality in, 197,199t
        case relevance in,
          197-198,199t
        case topics in, 198-201,200t
        descriptive results of,
          197-201,200t
        findings in, 203-208,205f

change entities in, 130-134,135f
development of, 129-134
quality in, 132
time-related changes in, 130
Television, "reality," 4-5
TERC, Inc., 112-113
Tharp, R., 192
The Cavalier Daily, 3
The Gallup Organization
*The Interplanetary Teacher Learning
    Exchange (TITLE),* 209
Theme(s), in development of
    sexual harassment cases
    using cognitive flexibility
    hypertext, 215-216
THES. *See* Times Higher
    Education Supplement
    (THES)
Thinking, critical, in interactive
    learning environments,
    support for, 17-32
Third-generation distance
    education, 48-49
Thomas, L., 84
Times Higher Education
    Supplement (THES), 70
TITLE. *See The Interplanetary
    Teacher Learning
    Exchange (TITLE)*
Tom, A., 86
Top Class, 151
Training
    informed, 259
    self-control, 260
Transfer of knowledge, in cognitive
    flexibility hypertext for
    developing sexual harass-
    ment cases, 222-224,
    223t,224t
Treahy, D., 107
Trentin, G., 47,80-81,84
Troubleshooting, issues associated
    with, 43-44

UCEA. *See* University Council for
    Educational Administration
    (UCEA)
United States Congress, anger directed
    at, 6
University Council for Educational
    Administration (UCEA), 251
University of Missouri-Columbia
    Center for Technology
    Innovations in Education,
    251,255

VanDoren, C., 18
Varimax rotation, 99
Vaughn, M., 27-28,28
Violence, in media, 4-5
Virtual-U, 234
Visscher, A., 133
Vygotsky, L.S., 21,92,201

Warner, M.M., 171
WebCT, 43
WebTeach, 152,153f,154-155,156-157
Wegerif, R., 244
Wenger, E., 110
Wideband CU-SeeMe internet
    solutions, 83
World Lecture Hall, 149-150
World Wide Web (WWW)
    communication tools of, in critical
        thinking, 23-28,25f. *See also*
        Critical thinking, Web com-
        munication tools in promo-
        tion of
    in education, asset vs. liability,
        1-16
    learning from, myths related to,
        159-169
        hyperlinking is good instruc-
        tion, 166-167

Milton Keynes UK
Ingram Content Group UK Ltd.
UKHW031135141024
449569UK00006B/167